TAKE HEART

TAKE HEART

CUT YOUR INHERITED RISKS OF HEART DISEASE

Edward D. Frohlich, M.D.,
and Genell J. Subak-Sharpe

CROWN PUBLISHERS, INC.   NEW YORK

Published by Crown Publishers, Inc., 201 East 50th Street,
New York, New York 10022. Member of the Crown Publishing Group.

CROWN is a trademark of Crown Publishers, Inc.

Manufactured in the United States of America

Library of Congress Cataloging-in-Publication Data
Frohlich, Edward D., 1941–
    Take heart: cut your inherited risks of heart disease
    / Edward D. Frohlich and Genell J. Subak-Sharpe.—1st ed.
        p.   cm.
    1. Heart—Infarction—Prevention. 2. Heart—Infarction—
Susceptibility. 3. Heart—Infarction—Risk factors. I. Subak Sharpe,
Genell J. II. Title.
RC685.I6F76   1990
616.1''2305—dc20   89-29025
ISBN 0-517-57172-2

Book design by June Marie Bennett

10 9 8 7 6 5 4 3 2 1

First Edition

This book is dedicated to our respective spouses, Sherry Frohlich and Gerald Subak-Sharpe, and to our children, Margie, Bruce, and Lara Frohlich, and David, Sarah, and Hope Subak-Sharpe. Their understanding, patience, and support have made this book possible.

CONTENTS

INTRODUCTION: THE NEXT REVOLUTION IN CARDIOLOGY

During my medical career, I have witnessed one of medical history's most profound revolutions: the mastery of many of the major forms of cardiovascular disease. First, medicine reversed the consequences of rheumatic, syphilitic, and congenital heart diseases. More recently, we have made tremendous inroads against high blood pressure, heart attacks, and strokes. As a result, the annual death toll from stroke is less than half what it was in 1972, and heart attack mortality is down by more than a third.

Many of these impressive newer gains are due to improved treatment of problems such as high blood pressure, elevated cholesterol, and coronary artery disease. But much of the success also stems from the public's remarkable interest in the new phenomenon of "wellness." While the war against cardiovascular disease is not yet over—it still remains our leading cause of death—we now stand poised at the beginning of another, perhaps even greater revolution: preventing most forms of heart disease from ever occurring. Our focus is not on any one risk factor; instead, it is on the total approach of an individual to a rational and balanced concept of wellness.

This book is intended to bring you to the forefront of this coming revolution by helping you formulate your own life plan to prevent a heart attack or stroke. But first, I should like to describe briefly a few of the medical events that have brought us to this new revolution—the era of preventive cardiology. Unlike prior successes that involved diagnosis and treatment, this one required the partnership of medicine and the public—or, more specifically, the doctor and patient.

I vividly remember the day that President Franklin Roosevelt died of a stroke—the "natural" (and in those days, all too common) consequence of progressive and unrelenting high blood pressure. During those last days of World War II there was no effective treatment for hypertension, and most of its victims died early in life from stroke, heart failure, or rapidly progressive "malignant" hypertension itself. Today, these virulent forms of hypertension are eminently treatable. And while most patients then were destined to have a premature death, this problem today has a bright future—provided that the physician and the patient with hypertension communicate with one another and work closely together.

When I was in medical school, we encountered diseases that are now rare. Hospitals were filled with people dying of heart failure caused by defective valves, the consequences of earlier childhood rheumatic fever. Another cause of heart failure, the long-term effects of syphilis, was also fairly common. Today, we very rarely see rheumatic failure, thanks to the widespread use of antibiotics against the strep infections of childhood. Similarly, antibiotics have dramatically lowered the incidence of syphilis-related heart disease.

In those earlier days we learned that high blood pressure

was a disease for which very little could be done. Today, a broad spectrum of effective drugs is available to treat it, and most people with high blood pressure can lead normal, productive lives. The same is true of hardening of the arteries, a condition called arteriosclerosis. Not that long ago, we thought it was an inevitable part of the aging process. Today, we know that this is not so; arteriosclerosis can be prevented, especially the form of the disease known as *athero*sclerosis, which is caused by a buildup of fatty deposits inside the walls of arteries.

Similarly, there was not much we could do back then about treating angina pectoris (chest pain), heart attacks, and other consequences of coronary artery disease. Nitroglycerine and digitalis were about the only drugs we had, and the side effects of both often limited their usefulness. The patient who survived a heart attack was destined to lead an invalid's life. In contrast, current therapy includes getting patients on their feet quickly; total approaches to physical rehabilitation, including exercise and open discussion of sexual activity; as well as a wide variety of drugs to relieve angina, to help prevent a subsequent heart attack, or to minimize further heart damage. Consequently, today's heart attack survivors are usually able to return to their work and continue to lead active and productive lives. But the most exciting news is that with sensible education, good patient-doctor communication, commonsense wellness techniques, diet, and medications to control weight, cholesterol, blood sugar, and pressure, it is now possible to prevent heart attacks in the first place.

In addition to these advances, in the 1960s open-heart surgery became feasible. Now, with new blood-bank technology and heart-lung pumps, we can replace or repair defective heart valves, bypass or open up clogged coronary arteries, and even replace badly diseased hearts with healthy ones. Operations also have been perfected to repair the hearts of newborn babies with congenital defects—babies who in the past would have died or lived very restricted lives.

The years since the end of World War II have been marked by advances that were unimaginable just a few decades earlier. Many of these exciting new developments should be credited to innovative research funded by the government's National Heart, Lung and Blood Institute, the American Heart Association, and the pharmaceutical industry. But even though these achievements in cardiovascular medicine have saved or improved millions of lives, we are only on the threshold of even more far-reaching changes that will carry us into the 21st century. Some involve deciphering the instructions programmed for us in our genes. But the remarkable thing is that many of these breakthroughs will not really be new, nor will they be confined to medicine (in the broadest sense). Instead, they will be related to, and dependent upon, the way we live, eat, exercise, and modify our behavior to deal with the stresses of day-to-day living.

In this book, you will learn that there is much that we can do to play out the hand of cards dealt to us by our genetic predisposition and our life-styles. Heart attacks and strokes are *not* a matter of fate or bad luck. Even if you are at increased risk for a heart attack, stroke, or other serious complications, you can improve your odds by following a practical and logical step-by-step approach to eliminating or minimizing risk factors. At the same time, you will be able to enjoy better health and a greater sense of well-being. In this approaching revolution against heart diseases, you can and will play a key role and an active one—and you can and will be able to reap the rewards.

1 WHAT'S YOUR RISK?

The term "risk factor" has now become part of the common parlance of both the medical profession and the general public. In fact, patients frequently come to their doctors to discuss their concerns over a specific risk factor. As a result, many physicians now emphasize the assessment and evaluation of risk factors, and their modification or reduction—including programs for seemingly healthy patients. This explains the "new" concept of "wellness" programs. Preventive maintenance is an accepted practice in industry; similarly, preventive cardiology is just as important in health care.

This emphasis on risk factors is relatively new. The term was coined in the early 1960s by Dr. William Kannel and his co-workers in the Framingham Heart Study. In fact, much of what we know about risk factors in general, and especially those for cardiovascular disease, comes from this landmark study, which has been going on for more than forty years. In the late 1940s, investigators headed by Dr. Kannel, enlisted several thousand residents of Framingham, a Boston suburb, for long-term analyses of their health. The objective was to identify specific factors that increase the likelihood for developing a subsequent heart attack, stroke, sudden death, heart failure, or other cardiovascular incident. Data began to appear by the late 1950s, and in a key paper published in 1960 dealing with Dr. Kannel's "Factors of Risk," he and his colleagues described the things that increased the likelihood of cardiovascular complications. Thus began the notion that, by altering some of these factors, we could prevent such catastrophic life-shattering events from happening. (It should be stressed that these risk factors apply to a number of diseases, not just heart attacks. In fact, it is pretty much the luck of the draw whether an individual with a number of the following risk factors will develop a heart attack, a stroke, or heart or kidney failure.)

UNAVOIDABLE RISK FACTORS

Framingham and other epidemiological studies in this country and elsewhere around the world have pinpointed some risk factors that are beyond our control. Specifically, these are:

Age. As might be expected, age increases the risk of a heart attack, stroke, or sudden death. Indeed, in most westernized (or, as termed by some, industrialized or acculturated) societies, blood pressure increases with age. As a result, about 55 percent of all heart attacks occur in people over the age of sixty-five; and 80 percent of those who die of a heart attack are sixty-five years or older.

Gender. By now, it is well known that men have a greater risk of heart attack than women. But this edge that women have over men lessens after the menopause. The female sex hormone estrogen is credited with this protective effect. After menopause, a woman's risk of a heart attack increases tenfold primarily because of the precipitous decrease in her body's ability to produce estrogen. Nevertheless, the attack rate never quite catches up with that of men, and recent studies indicate that women who take estrogen after menopause may continue to enjoy a lower incidence of coronary heart disease, all other factors being equal.

Heredity. People whose parents or other close relatives suffered early heart attacks (before the age of fifty) have an increased risk of heart attacks themselves. (This factor of genetic predisposition may one day come to be considered "modifiable," as our knowledge concerning gene manipulation increases; but that day is in the future.)

Race. Race is also a factor. In the United States, black people have a higher rate of certain cardiovascular diseases than whites. Native Americans also have higher incidences. The reasons for this are not fully understood, but likely clues are the prevalence of high blood pressure among the black population, and of overweight and diabetes mellitus among Native Americans.

AVOIDABLE OR MODIFIABLE FACTORS

The above four risk factors cannot be changed. But there are a number of others that can be avoided, controlled, or at least modified, which can reduce the risk of a heart attack. They include the following:

Cigarette smoking. The risk of heart attacks among cigarette smokers is more than double that of nonsmokers. The risk of sudden death—that is, death within the first hour of a heart attack—is two to four times greater for smokers than for nonsmokers. According to the most recent surgeon general's report on smoking and health, cigarette smoking is responsible for more than 200,000 heart attack deaths in the United States each year.

High blood pressure. Also known as hypertension, high blood pressure requires the heart to work harder. In order to deal with the increased pressure the heart eventually requires a larger pumping chamber. In time, this enlarged (hypertrophied) heart increases the risk of heart attack because the increased blood pressure and larger heart increase the heart muscle's demand for oxygen. People with high blood pressure also are at greater risk for sudden death, angina pectoris, stroke, kidney failure, and congestive heart failure. The last is a condition in which the heart can no longer pump enough blood, oxygen, and other nutrients to the body's organs. Fluid builds up in the lungs and other body tissues, so that the victim suffers shortness of breath and other symptoms of oxygen starvation.

High blood cholesterol. Cholesterol is a waxy substance that is essential to many vital body functions. When there is too much of it circulating in the blood, however, it becomes a major risk factor for the development of a heart attack. High blood cholesterol is linked closely to atherosclerosis—the buildup of fatty deposits in the artery walls. If the coronary arteries—the blood vessels that nourish the heart muscle—become clogged by cholesterol deposits, there is an enhanced risk of developing a heart attack. Severely narrowed coronary arteries also can lead to the chest pains characteristic of angina pectoris.

Diabetes mellitus. In diabetes, the body is unable to metabolize carbohydrates and other nutrients normally. The most common form of diabetes occurs in middle-aged overweight people. It may be present for many years without causing symptoms, but the high levels of blood sugar—the major characteristic of patients with diabetes—can be responsible for the many complications of the disease, including an increased risk of premature death. Diabetes also accelerates the process of atherosclerosis, thus raising the risk of heart attack.

Obesity. It has long been known that overweight people have more heart attacks than their normal-weight counterparts. We also know that the more you weigh, the greater is your cardiovascular risk. Obesity is usually defined as being more than 15 percent over your "ideal" or desirable body weight. More recently, studies have found that the distribution of the excess body fat is very important. Fat concentrated in the abdominal area—the so-called pot belly—is associated with an increased risk of a heart attack. Men are more likely to accumulate excess fat in the abdominal area, whereas women tend to store fat more in the buttocks and thighs (although this changes somewhat after menopause, when women, too, store more fat in the abdomen). You can tell if you have too much abdominal fat by comparing waist and hip measurements. A man's waist measurement should not exceed that of his hips; and a woman's waist should not be more than 80 percent of her hip measurement.

Alcohol. Consumption of more than one ounce of ethanol (or its equivalent) per day increases the risk of high blood pressure and stroke. Excessive alcohol consumption, especially in older people, also increases the risk of a heart attack, heart failure, and other complications.

There are other factors that have been linked to an increased risk of angina pectoris, heart attack, and sudden death, but they are not as clear-cut as those listed above. These include:

Sedentary life-style. A number of studies have found that people who are physically active tend to live longer and have a lower heart attack rate than those who are sedentary. But an association between exercise and heart attacks has not been proved. Some researchers believe that the impact of physical activity in the form of exercise on other risk factors may be more important than the direct effects of exercise itself. For example, physically active people are less likely to be overweight than their sedentary peers. Exercise can also help reduce blood cholesterol, and it seems to be important in controlling diabetes, perhaps through weight control.

Stress. It has long been observed that heart attacks often coincide with a stressful life event, such as the death of a loved one, a divorce, or a change in job. However, we do not know just what effects, if any, stress has on the heart. All of us are subjected to varying degrees of stress, and we all respond differently. It may be that the manner in which some people handle stressful situations makes them more vulnerable to heart attacks, but this too has not been proved.

Personality type. The relationship between personality and heart disease is also controversial. Some researchers have found that people with "Type A" personalities—who tend to be more aggressive, quick-tempered, driven, and overly time conscious—have more heart attacks than their calmer, more placid "Type B" counterparts. More recently, however, researchers have found that anger appears to be the most harmful of these personality characteristics, and that consistently angry, hostile people (for example, those who get angry when standing in line or hostile when tied up in traffic) have more heart attacks than less angry people who may have all the other Type A characteristics. This increased risk is believed to be due to hormonal factors.

MEASURING THE RISK: A CASE HISTORY

Paul Kimbal (not his real name) is a thirty-seven-year-old bank executive. His father had had his first heart attack at age thirty-six and had died when he had a second one at forty-two. Until now, Paul had been somewhat oblivious to his health and, aside from an occasional cold or other minor illness, he generally felt fine. But now he was worried—his thirty-nine-year-old brother had recently had a heart attack, and Paul was afraid that he would be next. He was referred to our clinic for an evaluation and counseling. (Incidentally, it is not unusual for patients to come to their physicians on the anniversaries of major illnesses that befell themselves or members of their families.)

Paul's physical examination showed the following:

■ Blood pressure—normal.
■ Blood cholesterol—in the borderline level of 230 milligrams per deciliter.
■ Weight—20 pounds over what is desirable (170 pounds) for his height, sex, age, and build.
■ Cigarette use—one pack a day.
■ Blood glucose—normal.

By his own admission, Paul showed many Type A personality characteristics: he was definitely achievement and career-oriented; he was very driven to succeed. "I'm a clock watcher," he said. "I can't stand to waste time or to be late." But he was also even-tempered: instead of getting angry over a delay or setback, he would work out a solution. He also took time out of his schedule to exercise: "I go to my health club during lunch at least three times a week," he explained. He also took work home most nights, and worked at least part of most weekends.

In talking with Paul, it emerged that he was convinced he was destined to have a heart attack, even though he felt fine and had no obvious symptoms. As a banker, he was used to working with statistics, and he wanted to know in precise terms just what his risk was. But he was also taking a fatalistic approach. "It's my wife who insisted I get a checkup," he revealed. "To my way of thinking, there's not much I can do one way or the other. When my card comes up and it says 'heart attack,' that's it. And I think my card is overdue. "

In calculating statistical risk, it's important to remember that risk is derived from studying large population groups, and consequently we can take a large group of people and predict that a certain percentage will have heart attacks. But given our present knowledge, it's impossible to predict with absolute accuracy whether or not any particular individual within that group is going to have one. Some people with numerous risk factors defy all odds and live long lives. The World War II British prime minister Winston Churchill was an example: he smoked cigars continuously, drank alcohol heavily, and was overweight, yet lived into his nineties. Then there are people who appear to be free of risk factors, but still suffer heart attacks at an early age. The best we can do is determine whether or not a person falls into a high-risk category, and if so, what can be done to better the odds.

Paul is a good example of a typical individual with un-avoidable risk factors: his gender and family history of early heart attacks. He also had some risk factors that could be eliminated, and by doing so, he could reduce his chances of becoming a heart victim. First we had to convince Paul that being born with certain risk factors did not mean that he was powerless to change his destiny as far as heart disease is concerned. The way he led his life would make a big differ-ence. Also, the likelihood of a heart attack increases tremendously with each additional risk factor. Thus, a man with a strong family history of heart attacks or premature death who smokes may increase his risk three to four times over what it would be if he didn't smoke. And if his cholesterol was high, his risk might be increased sevenfold.

So even though we could not promise Paul that he would not have a heart attack, we could tell him that if he quit smoking, lost a few pounds, and brought his blood cholesterol down to 200 milligrams per deciliter or less, his chances were going to be greatly improved.

CALCULATING YOUR OWN RISKS

In recent years, a number of researchers have developed special health-risk appraisals designed to help individuals calculate their own statistical risks. The American Heart Association has simplified these statistical appraisals into an easy self-assessment test (see Table 1, pages 14–17). This test covers the "big seven" risk factors that can be eliminated or controlled. If you score higher than 10, you have a moderate to high risk of a heart attack and you definitely should work at reducing it.

In subsequent chapters, we will discuss each of the risk factors in greater detail, along with specifics on how each can be eliminated or minimized. What worked for Paul Kimbal and countless others who may not have been born with the best of odds can work for you, too.

14

Table 1. The Heart Attack Risk Quiz

Use this table to find your total risk score.

FOR MEN

Systolic blood pressure
100 110 120 130 140 150 160 170 180 190 200

Enlarged left ventricle   No   Yes
Diabetes   No   Yes

POINTS   0 1 2 3 4 5 6 7 8 9 10

Note: Cigarette smoking is not a predictor of a heart attack for men

AGE

		36	38	40	42	44	46	48	50	55	60	65	70
T O T A L B L O O D C H O L E S T E R O L	165	3	6	9	11	14	16	18	19	23	26	27	27
	180	5	8	10	13	15	17	19	20	24	26	27	27
	195	7	9	12	14	16	18	20	21	24	26	27	27
	210	8	11	13	15	17	19	21	22	25	27	27	27
	225	10	12	15	17	19	20	22	23	26	27	28	27
	240	11	14	16	18	20	21	23	24	27	28	28	27
	255	13	15	17	19	21	23	24	25	27	28	28	27
	270	15	17	19	21	22	24	25	26	28	29	28	26
	285	16	18	20	22	24	25	26	27	29	29	28	26
	300	18	20	22	23	25	26	27	28	29	29	28	26
	315	20	22	23	25	26	27	28	29	30	30	29	26

ENTER POINTS FOR

Systolic blood pressure   _____
Enlarged left ventricle   _____
Glucose intolerance (diabetes)   _____
Age/cholesterol   _____

TOTAL RISK SCORE   _____

Now find your total risk score in the Probability section for men. Note: Probability is for men 35 to 70 years old.

Probability of a Heart Attack in the Next 6 Years

MEN

Total points	Probability★★	Total points	Probability★★
5	3	28	57
6	4	29	64
7	4	30	71
8	5	31	80
9	6	32	90
10	6	33	100
11	7	34	110
12	8	35	130
13	9	36	140
14	10	37	160
15	12	38	170
16	13	39	190
17	15	40	210
18	17	41	230
19	19	42	250
20	21	43	280
21	24	44	300
22	28	45	330
23	31	46	360
24	35	47	390
25	40	48	420
26	45	49	450
27	50		

★★Probability is your chance of having a heart attack based on 1000. For example, if you have a total of 10 points, your chances of having a heart attack in the next 6 years are 6 out of 1000. If you have 49 points, your chances jump 150-fold, to 450 chances in 1000.

Compiled by Erica Brittain, data from The Framingham Heart Study.

Use this table to find your total risk score.

FOR WOMEN

Systolic blood pressure

100	110	120	130	140	150	160	170	180	190	200

Cigarette smoking	No	Yes
Enlarged left ventricle	No	Yes
Diabetes	No	Yes

POINTS

0	1	2	3	4	5	6	7	8	9	10

AGE

TOTAL BLOOD CHOLESTEROL	36	38	40	42	44	46	48	50	55	60	65	70
165	0	2	4	5	7	9	10	12	15	18	20	21
180	1	3	4	6	8	9	11	12	16	18	20	22
195	2	3	5	7	9	10	12	13	16	19	21	22
210	3	4	6	8	10	11	13	14	17	19	21	22
225	4	5	7	9	10	12	13	15	17	20	21	23
240	4	6	8	10	11	13	14	15	18	20	22	23
255	5	7	9	11	12	13	15	16	19	21	22	23
270	6	8	10	11	13	14	16	17	19	21	23	24
285	7	9	11	12	14	15	16	17	20	22	23	24
300	8	10	12	13	15	16	17	18	21	22	24	24
315	9	11	13	14	15	17	18	19	21	23	24	25

ENTER POINTS FOR

Systolic blood pressure	_____
Cigarette smoking	_____
Enlarged left ventricle	_____
Glucose intolerance (diabetes)	_____
Age/cholesterol	_____

TOTAL RISK SCORE _____

Now find your total risk score in the Probability section for women.

Note: Probability is for women 35 to 70 years old.

Probability of a Heart Attack in the Next 6 Years

WOMEN

Total points	Probability**	Total points	Probability**
5	2	23	34
6	3	24	40
7	3	25	46
8	4	26	53
9	4	27	61
10	4	28	71
11	6	29	81
12	7	30	93
13	8	31	111
14	9	32	120
15	10	33	140
16	12	34	160
17	14	35	180
18	16	36	200
19	19	37	230
20	22	38	260
21	25	39	290
22	29	40	320

**Probability is your chance of having a heart attack based on 1000. For example, if you have a total of 10 points, your chances of having a heart attack in the next 6 years are 4 out of 1000. If you have 30 points, your chances jump 25-fold, to 93 chances in 1000. Compiled by Erica Brittain, data from The Framingham Heart Study.

2 TAKE A POSITIVE APPROACH

Now that you have a pretty good idea of your risk factors for a heart attack, the question is: What can you do about them? As was stressed in the previous chapter, most cardiovascular risk factors can be controlled or reduced, and the chapters that follow will offer specific recommendations for approaching each one. But before tackling individual factors, you should take an unbiased look at your life-style. You and only you can decide just how much that life-style is contributing to your heart attack risk, and how great your commitment will be to carrying out the necessary changes. This self-examination is probably the most important step you will take to lower your risk of a heart attack. If you find yourself unable or unwilling to deal with all the risk factors at once, then choose the most reasonable ones to tackle first. Having lowered the odds by reducing one or more factors of risk, a positive attitude will permit you to reassess those that you had deferred to a later time. The main objective is to maintain your positive approach by attacking just a few factors, or even one, at a time.

START WITH YOUR MIND-SET

In recent years, doctors and patients alike have taken a new and constructive look at the importance of mental attitude and outlook for improving health and overcoming disease. Health consciousness and a variety of wellness programs have gained popularity over the past decade, and we are now beginning to measure positive results in terms of improved health.

Norman Cousins in his widely read book *The Healing Heart* describes his heart attack and how, by taking charge with a positive attitude, he was able to put himself well on the way to recovery. He stresses that attitude is not a substitute for medical care, but an important, perhaps even vital, adjunct to it. He stresses that he learned how to "listen to his body," and was truly an informed partner in making important medical decisions.

In today's highly technological society, physicians (and the general public) often overlook this "power of positive thinking." Nevertheless, it is important to consider this aspect of a wellness program when one tries to come up with the reasons why some patients fare better than others. While the precise physiological mechanisms remain elusive, virtually every doctor can recall those patients who "made it" against seemingly impossible odds, whereas others who were not as ill or were given better odds at the outset, progressed in their illnesses or died despite superlative medical care. In looking for an explanation and common denominator, we are often left with vague concepts like "fighting spirit," "positive outlook," or "refusal to give up." Of course, there are cases in which even the staunchest determination and fiercest fighting spirit are not enough to prevail against those unrelenting factors of disease that make the odds unbeatable. Still, patients who demonstrate these qualities seem to have a very real and definite advantage over those who are more passive or willing to relegate their fate to physicians or other forces beyond their control. The important thing to remember is that, if you do not at least attempt to take these affairs into your own hands as you work with your doctor, no one else will. The decision, then, is yours. And the one factor that is so very important in insuring this success is a positive doctor-patient communication relationship.

LOOK AT THE POSITIVE SIDE

All too often, people faced with the need to alter their life-style take a negative viewpoint and look upon the changes as major sacrifices. We have all heard an overweight person moan, "I can't have anything that tastes like real food until I lose twenty pounds," or, "Dieting takes all the fun out of eating." We know the end result at the outset—no one wants to live a life of sacrifice. The dieter may give up favorite foods long enough to lost the 20 or 30 pounds, but chances are, as soon as the weight is lost, he or she will go back to the double scoops and heaping platefuls. In no time at all, the shed pounds are gained back, with maybe a few more added. And the sacrifices will start all over again.

The fact is, you don't need to approach weight loss with the conviction that you must "give up" anything, a basically negative concept. Your chances of success will be much better if you take a positive approach. For example: "I can still have my favorite foods—all I need to do is reduce the quantity and frequency." Once even a little success is achieved, the attainment may serve as positive feedback to proceed with your overall plan.

Remember, too, it is possible to reduce your risk even if you do not totally eliminate it. Moreover, there are no firm rules: you can arrive at your own priorities as to which risk factors you want to eliminate (for example, stop smoking, lower your blood pressure, decrease cholesterol, lose weight) and how to achieve these goals. Total correction of all risk factors obviously is best; correction or improvement of some factors is good, and no concern or action is deadly!

A similar litany of excuses prevails regarding exercise, stress management, stopping smoking, and other risk-factor reduction. So long as a life-style change is viewed as doing away with important pleasures, the chances of backsliding and failure are high. This alternative should be totally unacceptable to you; after all, didn't you decide to pick up this book? Let's accept the concept that winning at least *in part* will serve as a very important reinforcement factor. After all, this isn't the Super Bowl Game: you can be a winner even if your chances are only partially improved.

CHANGING THE ODDS: A CASE IN POINT

Fortunately, changing your heart attack risk factors can lead you to new, unexpected pleasures. The case of Jeff Allen, a fifty-one-year-old hospital administrator, comes to mind. Several months ago, Jeff suffered chest pains while helping his wife move furniture. The episode lasted only a few minutes, but was frightening nonetheless. A few days later, he again experienced chest pains—this time while walking up three flights of stairs in the hospital. He decided that it was time for a checkup to see if the pains were a warning sign of heart disease.

Jeff's chest pains were typical of angina pectoris, a condition that is invariably caused by coronary atherosclerosis, a narrowing of the arteries that supply blood to the heart muscle. But Jeff's physical examination revealed several other conditions that increased his risk of an early heart attack. For example, it turned out that he had mild high blood pressure. He was also about 30 pounds overweight. Questioning disclosed a number of life-style factors, including his diet, that further increased Jeff's risk. Like many New Orleans natives, he frequently had indulged his fondness for highly seasoned, fried foods, often in large quantities. He added a generous sprinkling of salt to his food before even tasting what was on his plate. His favorite pastime was watching sports on TV, usually with a beer and a bowl of salted nuts, potato chips, or pretzels nearby. He enjoyed socializing, and always went for the hors d'oeuvres set out with the drinks.

Examination showed that Jeff's blood pressure was only mildly elevated—in the range where a six-month trial of nondrug treatment, putting dietary restrictions on calories, alcohol, and sodium, was a reasonable first step to take. He and his wife met with a dietitian who explained the importance of losing weight, reducing alcohol consumption to levels of moderation, and restricting sodium intake.

"You mean I should start broiling or baking foods instead of frying them in butter?" Jeff's wife asked doubtfully. "And trim all the skin and fat off of chicken before cooking it?"

"But that's the best part!" cried Jeff. "And food without salt tastes like cardboard!"

The dietitian was prepared for this. "Bring me your favorite recipes," she replied, "and let's see what we can do to cut down on fat and sodium without ruining the taste or radically changing your diet."

Mrs. Allen voiced her doubts, but agreed to give it a try. She learned that not adding salt during food preparation and then using carefully measured quantities afterward would restrict total sodium intake. She also learned that with imaginative use of spices, herbs, and other flavorings, their favorite dishes could be turned into equally good heart-healthy foods. Jeff apparently liked what was served. Instead of breaded and fried chicken, he enjoyed a gourmet dish of skinless chicken breasts baked in a wine and mushroom sauce; instead of french fries, oven-browned potato crisps; and apple crisp topped with a cereal, raisins, and spices instead of apple pie à la mode.

Soon, a mill for freshly ground peppercorns replaced the salt shaker on the Allens' table. Fresh fruits, chili-flavored popcorn, and vegetable sticks with low-fat spicy dips replaced the high-salt, high-fat, and high-calorie snacks. Instead of spending so many hours watching TV, the couple began taking long walks on weekends and two or three evenings a week. Jeff started drinking soda water with lime or lemon at parties, or occasionally white wine, and found he could cut down on the hors d'oeuvres. One evening, he dropped in at a neighbor's to watch a football game. As he surveyed the coffee table laden with pretzels, nuts, and chips, he suddenly realized that they no longer tempted him. He actually preferred his new way of eating.

We also advised a program of moderate exercise conditioning to improve Jeff's endurance and help overcome his angina problems. To determine how much physical activity he could undertake without symptoms, Jeff was sent for an exercise stress test. Using the results of this test, we were able to work out a relatively simple exercise prescription. Jeff was instructed to walk at a brisk pace three or four times a week. In the beginning, he was told to walk for 15 minutes, and to stop if he felt short of breath or had chest pains. Every other week, he was to increase the time and distance covered until he could walk 2 miles in 30 minutes.

When Jeff returned for a checkup in three months, he was 10 pounds lighter and in good spirits. "I haven't felt this good in years," he confessed.

"And what about your diet?" he was asked.

"What diet?" he replied. "I'm eating better than ever."

Mrs. Allen echoed her husband's approval. "I'm learning a whole new approach to bringing out the best flavor in food," she said. "It was challenging and fun to modify my old recipes, and I know it's doing Jeff's heart good."

Eventually Jeff may need to take medication to lower his blood pressure. In the meantime, he's off to an excellent start in lowering his risk of a heart attack—and without ruining his life as he had feared would happen. Moreover, with this program he will probably require lower doses or fewer drugs.

In the following chapters you will read about other people who have reduced their risk factors and at the same time discovered an enjoyable new approach to living life at its fullest. By now it should be clear that this is not a book about self-sacrifice. Instead, it is intended to provide you with positive alternatives and advice on modifying your present life-style while at the same time increasing your chances of a longer and healthier life.

3 THE RISK OF CIGARETTE SMOKING

No matter what tobacco companies would like to have you believe, there is no longer any doubt that cigarette smoking is by far the number-one preventable cause of death in the United States. In his 1988 report on smoking and health, then Surgeon General C. Everett Koop, M.D., stressed: "The evidence establishing cigarette smoking as the single largest preventable cause of premature death and disability in the United States is overwhelming—totaling more than 50,000 studies from dozens of cultures. . . . It is estimated that smoking is responsible for well over 300,000 deaths annually in the United States." That's a staggering 15 percent of all deaths in this country. It outranks the combined total of deaths annually from AIDS, automobile accidents, homicides, and the other highly publicized causes of preventable death in this country. And Secretary of Health and Human Services, Louis W. Sullivan, M.D., indicated to Congress that the economic toll of illness, premature death, and related costs was in excess of $50 billion annually.

If you already are battling high odds of a heart attack, smoking can raise your risk even more. Many of my patients are surprised to learn this. They are well aware of the link between smoking and lung cancer, but many don't know that cigarette use also greatly raises the chance of a heart attack. In fact, many more people die of smoking-related heart attacks than of lung cancer and other pulmonary disorders put together. (It is of interest that the first person to relate cigarette smoking with lung cancer was the late Dr. Alton Ochsner, one of the founders of my institution, the Ochsner Clinic in New Orleans. He and his young associate, Dr. Michael DeBakey, reported this in the surgical literature more than fifty years ago, long before the first surgeon general's report on smoking.)

Risk factors interact with each other, so that the total risk imparted to a person by several factors is considerably more than the individual risks. Thus, by attacking smoking alone, your overall risk may be reduced by a factor far greater than simply the independent risk of smoking. Then if other factors, such as your weight or elevated blood pressure or high cholesterol, are also reduced, the total risk reduction is astounding.

However, helping smokers become ex-smokers is one of the more difficult tasks faced by physicians who would rather prevent a heart attack than treat one. The story of a patient of mine shows some of the problems that must be overcome. When I first saw Mark Lasky, he was forty-two years old and already could be described as a textbook candidate for a heart attack—he had almost all the risk factors. His father had died of a heart attack when he was only forty-nine. Mark had high blood pressure and was about 45 pounds overweight. Blood tests showed elevated levels of glucose—a sign of diabetes mellitus. His blood cholesterol level also was too high. These factors alone put him at tremendous risk for suffering a heart attack; and to make matters worse, he smoked more than two packs of cigarettes a day. His job as vice-president of a local construction contracting firm carried with it considerable stress and, by his own admission, he didn't cope very well with it.

"I lose my temper a lot," he confided, "and there are never enough hours in the day to get everything done."

Of course, Mark knew he was fighting heavy odds, and that is why he was seeking help. "I know I'm a medical mess," he said, "but I really want to turn my life around. I've got two young boys that I'd like to see graduate from college—something my dad never lived to see."

As I reviewed Mark's medical history and test results, I tried to formulate a plan of attack. I had to suggest a priority list for risk-factor reduction. Changing even one or two risk factors can be hard enough; turning around seven, as would be necessary in Mark's case, can be overwhelming.

Obviously, Mark could do nothing about his family history and the fact that he was male—two risk factor cards in the hand that he was dealt, and he had little choice but to play out his game of life with them. But he could do something with the other five factors—his elevated blood pressure, blood sugar, and cholesterol, his problem of overweight, and his cigarette smoking.

Very often, people like Mark try to jump in and correct a lifetime of poor habits all at once. It's akin to the long lists of New Year's resolutions that many of us make, only to fall back into our former patterns by the middle of January. Rather than load Mark down with more life-style changes than he could handle all at once, we decided it was best to tackle two of his risk factors first. So we put smoking at the head of the list. And since we could approach his high blood pressure problem with medication, without requiring his active participation in a weight reduction program, we also gave that a high priority. That way, Mark's major responsibility was to quit smoking, while mine was to select a treatment program to lower his blood pressure. If we could both do a good job in our respective areas, and he could begin to see the payoff in terms of feeling better, then we could move on to his other treatable risk factors, such as reducing his weight and bringing down his elevated blood sugar and cholesterol levels.

WHY DO PEOPLE SMOKE?

Make no mistake—kicking the cigarette habit is hard. As a former smoker myself, I know. But as more than 30 million ex-smokers in this country can attest, *it can be done!* About 95 percent of these former smokers managed to stop on their own. Quitting "cold turkey" is still the most popular method, but today there are many other approaches for those who can't simply stop overnight. If you fail in your first attempt, don't despair. About two-thirds of today's successful ex-smokers failed in their first attempts to quit. Some succeeded on their second tries; others required several attempts. But all of these people, by definition, succeeded in beating the odds associated with this insidious habit.

Millions of Americans share Mark's smoking history. Both of his parents were smokers, and he took up the habit when he was only thirteen. That may sound young, but carefully conducted studies have found that most smokers begin in their early teens. Also, children of parents who smoke are more likely to become tobacco users than are the offspring of nonsmokers. In fact, while the number of smokers is decreasing in this country, the number of smokers who are children and women is increasing at an alarming rate, which does not portend well for their future risk of heart disease.

People cite many reasons for smoking: to be a part of the crowd, to overcome feelings of nervousness, to have something to do with their hands, or for the pleasure it gives them. While these are the factors we use to explain the habit, they are only means of rationalization; the reason most smokers continue to use tobacco is that they are addicted to nicotine. Dr. Koop has frequently pointed out that cigarette smoking is an addictive habit just as powerful as cocaine. In plain terms, most people continue to smoke because they are hooked, physiologically dependent, on nicotine.

Here's how Mark described his addiction: "I wake up wanting a cigarette. Sometimes I light my first smoke of the day before even getting out of bed. And within minutes of finishing one cigarette, I begin to want another. If I put off lighting one, I begin to feel jittery. The first puff or two calms me down, and I can start thinking again."

Smokers commonly think that a cigarette has a calming or relaxing effect. Actually, nicotine is a powerful stimulant that increases stress or tension, rather than easing it. Within a few seconds of inhaling tobacco smoke, the nicotine reaches the brain, which in turn signals the adrenal glands to secrete catecholamines, principally epinephrine (adrenaline). These are the same hormones that are secreted as part of the body's reaction to stress (the so-called fight or flight response). Catecholamines speed up the heart rate and raise blood pressure. When a cigarette is finished, the effects of the nicotine wear off quickly and, as the "high" begins to wane, the person begins to want another cigarette, or dose of nicotine. This is a common characteristic of any addictive substance: once the body becomes accustomed to it, withdrawal of the substance will produce unpleasant symptoms that are relieved only by another dose.

Nicotine is not the only harmful substance in cigarettes. In fact, there are more than 4,000 chemical compounds in tobacco smoke, many of which are cancer-causing agents or poisons. In addition, with each puff, a smoker takes in large amounts of carbon monoxide. Carbon monoxide binds with the smoker's circulating red blood cells to form carboxyhemoglobin, decreasing the amount of oxygen available for uptake by the body's cells. To compensate, the heart must work even harder to deliver oxygen to the organs throughout the body. This is only one reason why smokers are so easily winded with even minimal physical effort.

Nicotine and other toxins in tobacco are detoxified in the liver, and, in time, they may lead to impaired liver function. One consequence is decreased activation of vitamin D, which in turn leads to impaired calcium metabolism. This may explain why many women who smoke are more vulnerable to osteoporosis (thinning of the bones) than nonsmokers. Some research also has implicated reduced calcium absorption as a factor in heart disease.

The tremendous increase in the number of women who smoke is also believed to be one factor in their rising incidence of heart attacks at an earlier age. In general, heart attacks are uncommon among premenopausal women, but after menopause, the incidence begins to go up. On the average, however, women who smoke experience menopause earlier than nonsmokers; and this might explain the rise in early heart attacks among women.

Most ex-smokers succeed by quitting cold turkey: they set a date for quitting, get rid of their cigarettes, and stop. Most people who do this experience at least a few days of withdrawal symptoms: jittery nerves, headache, inability to sleep, difficulty in concentrating, and as would be expected, extreme craving for a cigarette. Generally, the worst is over in a few days. But for some people, the withdrawal is simply too much to cope with and they give up. Mark had experienced this in prior attempts to stop, and didn't want to risk another failure.

HELP WITH QUITTING

Luckily, there are a number of new approaches for stopping smoking that are particularly helpful for people like Mark who are strongly addicted to nicotine. One entails the temporary use of nicotine gum, a prescription product that allows a smoker to break the habit without immediately removing the nicotine. The idea is to ease the transition from smoker to nonsmoker. After the person has stopped smoking, the nicotine gum is gradually tapered off.

There are other medications that an be used in the short term to ease a smoker through the withdrawal phase. One of these is clonidine, a drug which has generally been used to treat high blood pressure. Researchers at Columbia University in New York City have found that starting this medication a week or two before quitting and continuing it for four to six weeks thereafter can help smokers quit without experiencing withdrawal symptoms.

Still other approaches include hypnosis or joining a smoke-cessation program, such as those sponsored by the American Cancer Society, American Heart Association, Seventh-Day Adventist Church, or commercial groups such as SmokEnders. Some people stop by gradually tapering off, for example, by smoking one or two fewer cigarettes each day until they stop completely. Still others find that switching to a different brand helps them to quit more easily.

Saturation smoking is still another strategy practiced by many smoke-cessation clinics. It entails sitting in a small, enclosed room and smoking one cigarette after another until you can't face lighting up another. The idea is that the smoker will develop an aversion to smoking. While this works for some people, it certainly should not be recommended for anyone with heart or lung disease or for a person who is at a high risk for a heart attack. Indeed, the confines of the nonstop smoking room may place too great a strain on the heart and lungs as well as causing possible emotional trauma.

PLANNING FOR SUCCESS: ONE PATIENT'S STRATEGY

In Mark's case, we decided to use a combination of strategies. We started by working out a plan that was realistic and likely to succeed. He set a target date, to stop smoking in three weeks. This coincided with a slack period at his company so he would not have to contend with extra job stress superimposed upon the emotional rigors of smoke cessation. As part of his preparation for quitting, he agreed to switch to a menthol brand—not because it was any "safer" or better (so far as the heart is concerned, there's no such thing as a safe cigarette), but because he didn't particularly like them. Already he had found his own personal technique and additional motivation to reduce the pleasure of smoking.

Since Mark is very goal oriented, he made a deal with himself: if he succeeded in staying off cigarettes for six months, he would reward himself by buying a snazzy sports car, something he had wanted for years. If he took up smoking again, he would donate the money earmarked for his car to a scholarship fund. Granted, not everyone can afford such a lavish self-reward, but even a small reward can provide an added incentive to stop for good.

Like many people, Mark was worried that quitting would add to his weight problem. Smokers do tend to gain a few pounds after stopping. Food tastes better, so there may be a tendency to eat more. And metabolism may return to a normal, somewhat slower level, which may also lead to a gain in weight. Increased exercise provides an excellent counter to these changes: it burns up extra calories, and also helps control appetite. As an added plus, exercise has a calming effect (thought to be produced by the brain's release of endorphins and enkephalins, which are natural opiates) that can help overcome the jittery nerves that many people experience while quitting. Mark and his wife agreed to set aside a half hour or more every evening for a brisk walk.

I asked Mark to keep a smoking diary for a few days, taking the time to jot down the time and just what he was doing every time he smoked a cigarette (see Figure 1, page 34). Before his quitting date, we went over this log to spot the times when he would be most vulnerable. He already had described the need for his first cigarette shortly after waking. We also discovered that he always lit a cigarette when he had a cup of coffee, both during breaks and after meals. By substituting tea or a soft drink (even one with caffeine to give him the same "lift" as coffee), he could short-circuit this association of a cigarette and coffee. His evening walk provided an alternative to his usual after-dinner coffee and cigarette.

Mark also smoked while driving back and forth to work. This could be made more difficult by removing the ashtray and cigarette lighter from his car, and also by declaring the car a no-smoking vehicle, not only for Mark but also for his car-pool colleagues. Similarly, he bought a "Thank you for not smoking" sign for his desk and warned his colleagues that, as of his target quitting date, his office was strictly off limits for smoking, including cigars and pipes.

Finally, to provide extra peace of mind, he filled my prescription for six boxes of nicotine gum that he could use in case the withdrawal symptoms became too much to deal with. "I don't think I'm going to need it," he said, "but I'd like to know it's there just in case." In exchange for the gum,

Mark agreed to throw out all of his cigarettes and also to clear away ashtrays, matches, lighters, and all other smoking paraphernalia. Better the nicotine gum than a pack of cigarettes hidden away somewhere! This part of Mark's risk-factor war has a happy ending. He stuck to his stop-smoking target date. "I admit I had a few rough days," he said, "but I was determined to succeed this time." And he did, without even chewing one stick of the nicotine gum. "I didn't want to get hooked on that, too," he explained. "Luckily, I had enough other coping techniques all worked out and I really didn't need the gum." The last time I saw Mark, he was taking his nine-year-old son for a drive in a bright red sports car. And he's making similar progress in reducing his other risk factors. Before long, his odds of a heart attack should be no greater than for any other man his age with a family history of early heart attacks.

Figure 1. Mark's Smoking Diary

Time of Cigarette	Circumstance
7:00 a.m.	*Just got up*
7:30	*After shaving*
7:45	*With coffee, before going to work*
8:15	*Driving to work*
8:45	*With colleagues before work*
9:25	*Talking on phone*
10:00	*Coffee break*
10:45	*After meeting with boss*
11:30	*Needed to concentrate*
12:20 p.m.	*Waiting for lunch order*

Time of Cigarette	Circumstance
12:55	*With coffee after lunch*
1:15	*Driving to construction site*
2:00 and 2:20	*During meeting with job foreman*
2:45	*Felt need to smoke*
3:10	*Driving back to office*
4:00	*Late coffee break*
4:30	*Going over new contract*
5:30	*Driving home*
6:00	*With beer while watching TV news*
6:20	*Still watching TV*
6:45	*Waiting for dinner*
7:30	*With coffee and dessert*
7:45	*Second cup of coffee*
8:10	*Watching TV*
8:30	*Commercial break, with beer*
9:00	*Working on report for meeting*
9:20	*Same as above*
10:00	*Watching late news*
10:30	*With pretzels and cheese*
11:00	*Before going to bed*
11:45	*After sex*

Note: counted cigarettes left in pack—forgot to write down 6—all smoked during course of working day.

4 CONTROLLING HIGH BLOOD PRESSURE

When I first saw Mark Lasky, the patient described in the last chapter, in addition to his hereditary and life-style risk factors he had several medical problems that increased his risk of a heart attack. Foremost among these was his elevated blood pressure. He also had elevated levels of blood cholesterol and blood sugar. Although each of these risk factors is important, we had decided to start with the control of his high blood pressure through medication (while he himself was giving up smoking), after which we would work with him to lower his cholesterol and blood sugar through diet modification.

Today, most of the 63 million Americans with high blood pressure can lead long, productive lives free of the serious and dreaded complications of this disease. But this is a fairly recent development, and one of the most remarkable accomplishments in modern medicine. It has been my privilege to be a participant in this research and in the development of innovative treatments for high blood pressure.

When I was a medical student in the early 1950s, we were taught that there was little we could do about high blood pressure. Putting patients on a strict salt-restricted diet, like the regimen of fruit and rice proposed by Dr. Walter Kempner, helped, but not many could stick to such a difficult diet. And even among those who could, not all achieved lowered blood pressure. Then came a series of discoveries that led to the first antihypertensive drugs and dramatically improved the outlook for people with this disease.

Despite the many advances in both the detection and treatment of high blood pressure, however, many misconceptions persist about the condition. For example, Mark Lasky knew that his high blood pressure could be controlled by drugs, but as he said, when first referred to our clinic, "I've heard those medications are worse than the disease." Further questioning revealed his misconception that the drugs would either render him impotent or dull his mental functioning to the point where "I'd be some kind of zombie." Unfortunately, these notions are not that uncommon. Yet a better understanding of high blood pressure—or hypertension, to use its medical name—and its treatment will allay such fears.

WHAT IS BLOOD PRESSURE?

Each time your heart beats, it pumps a few ounces of blood into the aorta, the largest artery in the body. The body's circulatory system can be compared to a tree: the aorta has two major branch systems, one supplying blood vessels and their organs in the upper part of the body and the other, those in the abdomen and lower limbs. These large arteries branch off into smaller arteries going to specific body parts and organs, and the smaller arteries in turn feed into very small vessels called arterioles. The arterioles finally branch into

capillaries, which are microscopic blood vessels that deliver
oxygen and other nutrients to each of the billions of cells in
the body. The capillaries also collect waste from these cells,
and the blood, which by now has been depleted of its oxygen, begins the trip back to the heart and lungs. The
capillaries feed into tiny veins called venules, which unite
with other venules to form larger veins as the deoxygenated
blood travels back to the heart.

A certain amount of force or pressure is needed to keep
blood propelling through the body's vast network of some
60,000 miles of vessels. The amount of force exerted against
the artery walls to maintain this flow is referred to as "blood
pressure." This pressure is not steady, as is water pressure
when it flows through a faucet or hose. Instead, it comes in
spurts or waves, which are determined by the heart's beating
or pumping action. The force against the arterial walls is
highest when the heart muscle contracts to force blood into
the aorta. This is called the "systolic" or pumping pressure.
The pressure is at its lowest when the heart is resting between
beats and filling with blood in preparation for the next beat.
This is called the "diastolic" or resting pressure. When your
examining doctor uses two numbers to record your blood
pressure—for example, 120 over 80—the first number is the
systolic pressure and the second, the diastolic.

Blood pressure is usually measured with an instrument
called a sphygmomanometer, which consists of an inflatable
cuff, tubing, and a column of mercury. The cuff is wrapped
around your arm, and inflated until it is tight enough to halt
the flow of blood through the artery running down the inside
of your arm. A stethoscope is placed over the artery and air is
released from the cuff to allow the blood flow to resume. The
height of the mercury column when the first sound of rushing blood occurs is the systolic pressure. The cuff is deflated
further, and when the sound of rushing blood disappears, the

diastolic pressure is recorded. (More modern sphygmoma-nometers use a dial or digital device instead of a mercury column.) The resulting measurement of systolic and diastolic blood pressure is expressed in millimeters of mercury. Thus, a reading of 120 millimeters of mercury over 80 millimeters of mercury would be abbreviated as 120/80 mmHg, Hg being the symbol for mercury.

Over the course of a day, your blood pressure can fluctuate widely. Normally, it is lowest when you are sleeping. It begins to rise in the early morning hours, just before you wake, and will rise or fall during the course of the day in response to various activities. For example, blood pressure rises when you exercise because your muscles demand extra oxygen. It also goes up when you are confronted by a stressful situation—part of the body's fight or flight response. These normal fluctuations generally are not important clinically: high blood pressure becomes a medical problem only when it is sustained at abnormally high levels. That is why several blood pressure readings taken at different times are needed to establish a diagnosis of high blood pressure.

Until recently, even doctors disagreed as to what constitutes high blood pressure or hypertension. Today, however, we have standard guidelines, developed by the National High Blood Pressure Education Program, for both the diagnosis and treatment of high blood pressure (see Table 2, page 40). To establish a diagnosis of hypertension, blood pressure is measured two or more times and these readings are averaged. If the average is consistently elevated on three different occasions, a diagnosis of high blood pressure, which may be classified as mild, moderate, or severe, is established.

Table 2. Classification of Blood Pressure in Adults Over the Age of 18

Range (mmHg)	Classification
DIASTOLIC	
Below 85	Normal
85–89	High normal
90–104	Mild hypertension
105–114	Moderate hypertension
115 and greater	Severe hypertension (when diastolic pressure is less than 90)
SYSTOLIC	
Below 140	Normal
140–159	Borderline isolated systolic hypertension
160 and greater	Isolated systolic hypertension

Established by the National High Blood Pressure Education Program, 1984, National Heart, Lung and Blood Institute

CONSEQUENCES OF HIGH BLOOD PRESSURE

High blood pressure is often called the "silent killer" because it can exist for years without causing any obvious symptoms. But even if there are no symptoms, an elevated pressure can cause serious damage to the blood vessels, heart, and kidneys. Untreated high blood pressure also can damage the tiny blood vessels in the eyes. In fact, by examining these blood vessels with an ophthalmoscope—an instrument that shines a light into the eyes and enables us to look at the arteries through a magnifying device—we can gauge the degree of constriction of the blood vessels in the eyes, and by inference, of the kidneys and elsewhere in the body.

Some organs are especially vulnerable to damage from high blood pressure. These "target organs" include:

The blood vessels. The arteries are effected by hypertension in two ways. The smaller arteries constrict as a result of the hypertensive disease, thereby offering a greater resistance to the forward flow of blood as it is propelled by the heart's contraction. In time, the walls of these narrowed blood vessels become thicker, which in turn necessitates greater pressure in order to permit continued flow of blood.

The second effect of hypertension on the blood vessels involves the development of arteriosclerosis, or hardening of the arteries. Fatty deposits collect along the walls of these damaged arteries, a process called atherosclerosis. Hypertension accelerates this atherosclerotic process. The coronary arteries, which nourish the heart muscles, are particularly vulnerable to atherosclerosis. A heart attack occurs when one of these narrowed arteries becomes blocked, either by a fatty deposit or a clot at the site of narrowing. The carotid artery, and other arteries that carry blood to the brain, may become narrowed or blocked by arteriosclerosis, leading to an occlusive stroke. High blood pressure may promote a rupture of the vessels *in* the brain, causing a hemorrhagic stroke. Blood vessels in the legs sometimes become narrowed or clogged, resulting in decreased circulation to the lower legs and feet, and pain when walking.

The brain. Sustained high blood pressure can weaken one or more of the tiny blood vessels in the brain. (The ballooning out of one of these weakened vessels is called an aneurysm.) A hemorrhagic stroke results when an aneurysm ruptures and bleeds. Instead of bursting, a diseased blood vessel may be narrowed or clogged. This, too, can cause a stroke. A condition produced by constriction or temporary blockage to the brain is called transient ischemic attacks or TIAs. These are ministrokes that may cause temporary paralysis or loss of function. A TIA is often a prelude to a full-blown stroke. Repeated ministrokes also can cause a loss of mental function called multi-infarct dementia, which can be mistaken for Alzheimer's disease.

The heart. High blood pressure forces the heart to work harder. The heart is made up mostly of muscle (the myocardium); and like any other muscle, it enlarges in response to extra exercise. This enlargement of a heart chamber (the left ventricle) is called hypertrophy. Development of left ventricular hypertrophy is an independent risk fact for a heart attack, probably as a result of its increased instability (producing unusual heartbeats) and insufficient blood supply for such a large mass of muscle. Eventually, this enlarged heart muscle weakens and can no longer keep up with the needs of the body for blood supply. This causes a backup of fluid in the heart and lungs, a condition called congestive heart failure.

The kidneys. The kidneys contain millions of tiny units called nephrons, which filter wastes from the blood. High blood pressure can damage these nephrons, thereby reducing the kidney's ability to filter the blood. In time, this can cause serious kidney damage and even renal (kidney) failure. In fact, high blood pressure, especially if it is complicated by diabetes, is the most common cause of chronic kidney failure in the United States.

The eyes. Long-term high blood pressure can damage the tiny blood vessel's in the eye, leading to a loss of vision.

Usually, these potentially serious consequences of high blood pressure take many years to develop to the point where they cause symptoms. That is why high blood pressure is such an insidious disease: even though there may be no symptoms, it is silently causing damage, often irreparable, to vital organs. Very often, the first symptom will be a heart attack or stroke. Obviously, it is far better to detect and treat the disease before it reaches such a critical stage.

CAUSES OF HIGH BLOOD PRESSURE

Normally, blood pressure is controlled through a complex interplay of many factors involving the body chemistry. These control mechanisms can go awry in numerous ways, and as a result, there is no single identifiable cause of high blood pressure in the large majority (90 to 95 percent) of people with hypertension. This type of high blood pressure is called primary or essential hypertension. In essence, it is a disease of blood pressure regulation.

In some cases, the high blood pressure is a result of some other medical condition; this is referred to as secondary hypertension. Kidney disorders are the most common causes of secondary hypertension. Hormonal imbalances can also cause high blood pressure, but these are rare. Sometimes hypertension may be produced or worsened by certain foods, chemicals, or drugs, for example, excessive alcohol (more than an ounce a day), certain types of nose drops or cold pills, birth control pills, steroid medications, some of the nonsteroidal anti-inflammatory drugs (used to treat arthritis), and street drugs, most notably cocaine. In some cases of secondary hypertension, treating or removing the underlying cause will cure the blood pressure problem.

In the 90 to 95 percent of patients whose high blood pressure has no apparent cause, heredity seems to be the major factor. We have long known that high blood pressure often runs in families. Blacks are about twice as likely as whites (40 versus 20 percent respectively) to have the disease. Other inherited disorders, such as diabetes and perhaps obesity, are strongly linked to high blood pressure. In some hypertensive people who are overweight or who have diabetes, losing excess weight may be all that is needed to normalize both blood pressure and diabetes.

As noted, a high-salt (or more specifically, sodium) diet is linked to high blood pressure. However, contrary to popular belief, excess salt per se does not cause hypertension except in people with a (probably inherited) trait that allows sodium to raise blood pressure. Since a large number of Americans have this trait, the American Heart Association urges that we all cut down on sodium intake to less than 3.0 grams per day.

TREATMENT OF HIGH BLOOD PRESSURE

In 1972, when the Joint National Committee on Detection, Evaluation and Treatment of High Blood Pressure was formed, there were three major classes of medications to lower blood pressure. These were:

Thiazide diuretics. Diuretics, or water pills as they are commonly called, work by increasing excretion of sodium and water from the body via the kidneys, thereby lowering blood pressure by reducing sodium and the volume of fluids in the body. They are among the oldest of the antihypertensive drugs; chlorothiazide and hydrochlorothiazide, which are still the prototype thiazide diuretics, were first introduced in 1958.

Vasodilators. These drugs work by widening (dilating) the arterioles, the tiny arteries that control blood pressure. This is accomplished by relaxing the smooth muscles that encircle the walls of the arterioles. Blood pressure rises when the arterioles are constricted and falls when they are more relaxed and dilated. One of the first effective antihypertensive drugs—hydralazine—was a vasodilator. It was developed in Switzerland and first given to a patient in the United States in 1951. It has remained an important drug ever since.

Adrenergic inhibitors. These drugs act through inhibiting the autonomic nervous system to reduce the nerve control of the heart and blood vessels and also by dilating the arterioles. Within this category of drugs, there are specific medications that work on different sites. For example, the adrenergic inhibitors most used today are prazosin and other drugs that block the alpha receptors on the arterioles' smooth muscle walls, causing the arterioles to dilate and thereby lowering blood pressure.

Older, less commonly used drugs in this category include the centrally acting adrenergic inhibitors (methyldopa, clonidine, and others), which lower blood pressure by causing alpha receptors in the brain to reduce their outflow of impulses to the heart and blood vessels. The ganglionic blocking drugs (reserpine, guanethidine, and others) are very powerful inhibitors of both the sympathetic nerves that constrict blood vessels as well as the parasympathetic nerves that have other functions. As a result, these medications lower blood pressure, but they also have other undesirable side effects that have limited their use, as other medications with fewer side effects became available.

Although most of these older drugs still have a place in the treatment of high blood pressure, they also have major drawbacks. A diuretic alone often will reduce mild to moderate hypertension to within normal ranges, but it may also have a number of potential side effects. Thiazide diuretics increase the body's excretion of potassium—not just sodium—and this can upset the body's biochemical, or electrolyte, balance. Diuretics can also raise blood levels of uric acid, which can bring on an attack of gout; glucose, which can worsen diabetes; and of cholesterol. Some people who take diuretics become less tolerant to sun, which can lead to rashes and sunburn. They also may cause impotence, which has prompted some men to stop taking blood pressure medications.

In time, adrenergic blockers and some of the vasodilators cause the body to retain fluid, so unless they are taken with a diuretic, they are not effective in long-term control of high blood pressure. They, too, have a variety of side effects. Many of these problems have been eliminated or minimized by the development of newer classes of antihypertensive drugs. These include:

Beta adrenergic inhibitors (beta blockers). These drugs have been used in the United States for more than twenty years, but they were originally introduced for the treatment of angina and cardiac arrhythmias. In the early 1970s, they were approved for the treatment of high blood pressure. There are many different beta blockers; propranolol was the first to be used in this country and is still widely prescribed.

Beta blockers act through inhibiting the autonomic nervous system, but more specifically, they act on the sympathetic or adrenergic components. They work by slowing the heart rate, reducing the amount of blood that is pumped with each beat, and lowering the heart's need for oxygen. That is why they are effective in relieving the chest pains of angina in patients with coronary artery disease. About half of patients with mild to moderate hypertension can be effectively treated with beta blockers alone; other people may use them in combination with a low dose of a diuretic or other blood pressure–lowering medication. For reasons that are not fully understood, when they are used alone, these drugs seem to work better in white people than in black. Most people tolerate them well, but in some cases they can cause unusual tiredness, depression, nightmares, and sexual problems. People with asthma, emphysema, heart failure, or a heart condition in which there is a blockage of normal electrical impulses should not take beta blockers.

Angiotensin converting enzyme (ACE) inhibitors. These are among the two newest groups of antihypertensive drugs. These drugs work through the body's complex renin-angiotensin-aldesterone system. The kidneys are especially important in regulating blood pressure. Renin, an enzyme that is secreted by the kidneys, prompts the formation of a substance called angiotensin I. As this substance passes through the body's circulation, it forms angiotensin II, which is one of the body's most potent chemicals that raises blood pressure. Angiotensin II raises blood pressure by causing the muscles in the arteriole walls to constrict and also by stimulating the adrenal glands to secrete a hormone called aldesterone, which also raises blood pressure.

ACE inhibitors work by blocking the enzyme that converts angiotensin I to angiotensin II. They may be taken alone or along with a diuretic, which increases their effectiveness. Captopril was the first ACE inhibitor; several others, including enalapril and lisinopril, are now available. They have fewer side effects than older antihypertensive drugs. The most common are rashes (in 4 to 7 percent of patients), cough (3 to 5 percent), itching (2 percent), loss of taste (2 to 4 percent), and swelling of the face, mouth, or legs (less than 1 percent).

Calcium-channel blockers or calcium antagonists. Small amounts of calcium circulate constantly in the blood and are necessary for muscle contraction. For example, without calcium, the heart would be unable to beat. Calcium also is used by the tiny muscles encircling the arterioles to constrict, thereby raising blood pressure. When these muscles relax their tone, the arterioles widen or dilate, and blood pressure falls. Calcium blockers work by blocking the entry of some calcium into the muscle cells, thereby causing them to relax or dilate. Verapamil, nifedipine, and diltiazem were the first of the calcium-channel blockers; recently, several more have been introduced. They were first used to treat chest pains related to coronary spasms and angina, but today they are widely used to treat high blood pressure as well.

As with ACE inhibitors, calcium blockers tend to have few serious side effects. The most common are constipation, hypotension (excessive lowering of blood pressure), dizziness, swelling, and cardiac arrhythmias. They should not be used by patients with certain types of arrhythmias or heart failure.

Today's variety of antihypertensive medications allow doctors to tailor the treatment to the individual patient. And new classes of blood pressure-lowering properties are being developed at this time that are very specific in action and, hopefully, with still less side effects. When the first blood pressure–lowering drugs were introduced, we were content with simply lowering the elevated blood pressure, even if there were uncomfortable side effects. After all, we reasoned, you can live with certain side effects if doing so will help you avoid a heart attack, stroke, or other life-threatening complications. And initially, we prescribed therapy mostly for patients with the more severe degrees of hypertension. Now, with medications that have fewer side effects, we are able to treat patients with less severe hypertension in order to prevent its progression. The benefits derived from treatment far outweigh the costs, discomfort, or side effects of the medications.

Moreover, as we have gained experience in treating high blood pressure, we are better able to select effective medications that are most likely to work with the fewest side effects in specific groups of patients. For example, we know that beta blockers work particularly well in young patients who have more forceful and rapid heartbeats than older people. ACE inhibitors and calcium antagonists are not as likely to cause sexual dysfunction as diuretics, adrenergic inhibitors, or beta blockers. And they do not have the metabolic side effects associated with some of the older drugs. Moreover, they also may be used in combination therapy to reduce the dosages and side effects encountered with other drugs.

OTHER APPROACHES TO TREATMENT

Even though drug therapy has revolutionized the treatment of high blood pressure, it is by no means the only approach to controlling the disease. Life-style changes also are instrumental, and indeed, there are a number of patients whose blood pressure can be controlled—at least for a time—without any medication. The latest guidelines from the National High Blood Pressure Education Program suggests that, for patients with mild to moderate high blood pressure (those whose diastolic readings are 90 to 95 mmHg), non-drug treatment may be tried for three to six months. This entails altering certain habits or life-style factors that may contribute to your high blood pressure.

Reduce your salt intake. Perhaps a third of Americans with high blood pressure may be sensitive to sodium. A high-sodium diet may contribute to their high blood pressure whereas cutting back on sodium may help reduce it. Black Americans tend to be more sodium sensitive than whites in this country; they also tend to consume more salty foods, which may partly explain their increased incidence of high blood pressure.

Sodium and chloride, which make up ordinary table salt, are essential to maintain life, but only a very small amount is needed. The typical American diet contains upward of 20 grams of salt a day, many times what we actually need. About half of this sodium comes from processed foods, where it is used as a preservative, flavoring, or color enhancer. The remainder is added in cooking or at the table. In addition, many foods naturally contain varying amounts of sodium; you will get plenty even if you never add any salt to food at the table or when cooking. In fact, most people who are trying to cut their sodium intake start with reducing the amount of salt used in cooking and at the table. In our household, we've found that little or no salt is needed in food preparation: spices and herbs add all the flavor that is needed. The same goes for adding salt at the table.

For most people, it's the canned, frozen, and processed as well as the restaurant foods that are the big problem areas. Many processed foods contain large amounts of salt, including cereals, soft drinks, and other items that taste sweet instead of salty. (Table 3, pages 51–53, lists foods that are especially high in salt.) If you are trying to reduce your salt intake, learn to check labels for key words. Don't be misled by terms like "light" (or "lite") or "low-sodium." These simply mean that the food contains less salt than ordinary; it still may have more than you need or want. Remember, too, that in checking labels, the key word is not necessarily "salt"; look also for "sodium" or "soda." Many ingredients like baking soda, sodium bicarbonate, or monosodium glutamate (MSG) contain large amounts of sodium.

Sometimes salt can be washed out of processed foods. For example, regular canned tuna fish is very high in sodium. If you buy water-packed tuna, drain off and discard the water, and then rinse the tuna itself under cold, running water, you can remove a good deal of the salt. Canned and frozen vegetables also can be rinsed to remove salt.

Eating out can pose special problems to anyone on a sodium-restricted diet. Fast foods also tend to be loaded with salt (as well as fat), but even salad-bar items may have added salt, MSG, or other sources of sodium. When eating out, try to go to the same restaurants regularly, where the food is prepared to order, and ask that your meal be cooked without added salt or MSG. One patient of mine, for example, was able to persuade the chef at his favorite restaurant to prepare his soup with a special low-salt stock.

Table 3. Sodium Content of Selected Foods

Food	Portion	mg. of Sodium
MILK AND DAIRY PRODUCTS		
milk, fresh	1 cup	120
American cheese	1 ounce	320
cheddar cheese	1 ounce	195
cottage cheese (1%–2% fat)	1 cup	920
Swiss cheese, American-made	1 ounce	200
butter (salted)	1 tablespoon	125
margarine	1 tablespoon	150
yogurt, plain, low-fat	1 cup	160
MEATS, POULTRY, AND FISH		
bacon	1 strip	765
bologna	1 slice	365
Canadian bacon	1-ounce slice	385
corned beef	3 ½ ounces	1740
herring, smoked	3 ounce	5235
mussels	3 ½ ounces	290
tuna, canned in water	6 ½ ounces	865
tuna, canned in oil	6 ½ ounces	1160
salmon, canned	2 ½ ounces	350
CANNED AND PROCESSED VEGETABLES		
canned soups	1 can	1900–2460
asparagus	6 spears	270
beans, green	½ cup	270
corn, kernels	1 cup	590

Food	Portion	mg. of Sodium
mixed vegetables	1 cup	505
peas	¾ cup	235
spinach, frozen	½ cup	350

GRAIN PRODUCTS

saltines	2 crackers	65
Ritz crackers	3 crackers	95
soda crackers	2 crackers	155
rye bread, American	1 slice	130
white bread	1 slice	115
whole wheat bread	1 slice	120
corn bread	1 slice	220
Italian bread	1 slice	120
honey wheatberry bread	1 slice	160
sourdough break	1 slice	155

CEREALS

All-bran	½ cup	410
Corn flakes	1 cup	290
Grape-nuts	1 ounce	190
Raisin bran, Kellogg's	1 cup	290
Raisin bran, Post	1 cup	440
Cheerios	1 ¼ cup	305
Corn Bran	⅔ cup	240
Wheat Chex	⅔ cup	190
Wheat flakes	1 cup	350

SNACKS

pickles, dill	1 large	1430
peanuts, roasted	1 ounce	130
potato chips	1 ounce	210
cheese twists	1 ounce	330
cheese puffs	1 ounce	370

Food	Portion	mg. of Sodium
DESSERTS		
ice cream	1 cup	75–82
angel food cake	1 piece	160
cheesecake	1 piece	190
oatmeal cookies	2 large	260
cherry pastry	1 pastry	100
CONDIMENTS AND COOKING AIDS		
ketchup	1 tablespoon	160
soy sauce	1 tablespoon	860
teriyaki sauce	1 ounce	1150
Worcestershire sauce	1 teaspoon	50
baking powder	1 teaspoon	340
baking soda	1 teaspoon	820
bouillon cubes	1 cube	7715
garlic salt	1 tablespoon	1850
meat tenderizer	1 teaspoon	1745
salt	1 teaspoon	1955

Lose excess weight. Many hypertensive patients are overweight, and if this applies to you, gradually shedding those extra pounds may be all that is needed to bring down your blood pressure. (See Chapter 6 for more specific guidelines.)

Increase your exercise. Studies at Duke University Medical Center have found that exercise conditioning can reduce mild to moderate high blood pressure in some patients. While exercise alone may not be enough to normalize your high blood pressure, it has a number of important benefits that improve overall health. For example, exercise helps people achieve long-term weight control. Regular aerobic exercise reduces the heart's workload by increasing the body's efficiency in using oxygen. And exercise relieves tension and promotes a feeling of well-being. (See Chapter 8.) If you do suffer from high blood pressure, however, you should consult your doctor before undertaking any exercise program.

Limit your intake of alcohol. Consuming large amounts of alcohol (more than an ounce of ethanol a day) may contribute to high blood pressure. Studies have found that even a moderate consumption of alcohol (more than a glass of wine, a beer, or a mixed drink a day) increases the risk of stroke and raises blood pressure in proportion to the amount consumed. A prudent approach would be to limit alcohol consumption to these amounts or less.

Stop smoking. This is one positive action that cannot be overemphasized. As stressed in Chapter 3, smoking is by far the major cause of preventable death in the United States. If you have high blood pressure and smoke, your risk of a heart attack increases four- to fivefold what it would be if you did not smoke and did nothing about your pressure. Obviously, your high blood pressure should be treated, but if you smoke, your number-one priority should be to stop. Even if the blood pressure is well controlled, smoking may nullify the protective action against stroke. (See Chapter 3 for specific suggestions on how to go about quitting.)

Meditation, biofeedback, hypnosis, and other alternative treatments. Some of these strategies produce a temporary lowering of blood pressure, and may also have other benefits, such as improved techniques for coping with stress. While there may be considerable popular appeal to "natural" treatments, as opposed to the use of medications, none are considered reliable alternatives to more established treatments of high blood pressure.

Fad diets and treatments. Patients frequently ask me about vitamins, minerals, or special diets to control their high blood pressure. Good nutrition is important to maintaining health, but there is no magic dietary cure for this disease. Whenever I go abroad, I am struck by the advertisements in even reputable magazines for questionable remedies promising a quick cure for high blood pressure (and any number of other ills). These include drinking large amounts of garlic juice, taking high doses of vitamins, calcium, and other minerals, or drinking special waters. Some studies have found that very large amounts of garlic will reduce blood pressure. A little garlic as a flavoring can be marvelous, but few people (and those around them!) can tolerate the amounts advocated by some to control high blood pressure—an assertion that has never been proved scientifically. There is also no scientific evidence that large doses of calcium or any other mineral or vitamin will control the condition. In short, be suspicious of any fad diet or other unproved treatment of high blood pressure. Remember the old adage: If it sounds too good to be true, it probably is!

LIFELONG TREATMENT

Although the large majority of patients with primary hypertension can achieve satisfactory control of their high blood pressure, we still do not have a cure for the disease. Thus, treatment must be for life. This is not as onerous as it sounds: most people can get by on one or two drugs taken once or twice a day.

There are instances in which patients have been able to reduce their medication and keep their blood pressure under control. Studies have found that a few can even stop the medication entirely, but in many of these patients, their blood pressure gradually creeps back up to former levels (or even higher), and medications must be reinstituted. Life-style measures like smoke cessation, regular exercise, weight control, moderate sodium restriction, and alcohol moderation can improve blood pressure control and often allow patients to reduce the amount of medication needed. If you have high blood pressure, regular follow-up— usually three or four times a year—once your doctor has found a regimen that works for you, is essential. Home monitoring of your blood pressure also may be useful. A number of easy-to-use, relatively inexpensive home blood pressure machines are now available. The most reliable are those that use a column of mercury or a calibrated aneroid device. Unless the electronic digital devices are carefully calibrated, I do not recommend their use. Ask your doctor to show you how to take your own blood pressure, and when you go for a checkup, take your home device along with you to make sure that it produces the same blood pressure reading as the sphygmomanometer that your doctor uses.

In the first half of this century, a diagnosis of high blood pressure all too often was akin to a sentence of early death. Today, however, such a diagnosis calls for positive action but does not preclude living a full, productive life—with a greatly reduced risk of heart attack.

5 LOWERING YOUR CHOLESTEROL

Over the last twenty years, medical researchers have been amassing ever stronger evidence linking high levels of cholesterol circulating in the blood to an increased risk of heart attacks and premature death. Indeed, high cholesterol and obesity constitute the third largest cause of early death in the United States, right after high blood pressure and tobacco consumption.

The federal government's latest National Health and Nutritional Examination Survey (NHANES II) showed that one out of every four Americans over the age of twenty had cholesterol levels in the high-risk range (more than 240 milligrams per deciliter). Another 30 percent were in the borderline high-risk group (between 200 and 239 mg/dl). This is better than one of every two people in our country. Clearly, controlling serum cholesterol levels is crucial in our total approach to reducing the risk of an early heart attack and cardiovascular death.

Perhaps more than any other industrialized population, Americans worry about their cholesterol levels, a concern that is reflected in major changes in our diet and food-buying habits. Food manufacturers have responded positively to this threat by promoting a wide range of foods as being "cholesterol free." Unfortunately, some of this anti-cholesterol campaign has resulted in a good deal of confusion and misinformation about cholesterol. Moreover, until recently, even doctors have disagreed as to when high cholesterol should be treated. In all fairness, it should be noted that only recently have we had enough useful information to be able to arrive at a reasonable and meaningful consensus on cholesterol.

WHAT IS CHOLESTEROL?

Although most people talk and worry about cholesterol, I've found in talking to my patients that not many really know what it is and what it does. So let's start with a brief description of cholesterol as a natural body chemical. Cholesterol is a lipid, a family of many different compounds that share one major characteristic: they are insoluble in water. Lipids are generally classified as being simple, compound, or derived. But even within these general groups, there are many subgroups, and cholesterol falls into a subgroup of simple lipids that are waxlike alcohols.

In view of all the negative publicity about cholesterol, many of my patients are surprised to learn that its presence in the body is absolutely essential to maintain life. Almost every cell in your body contains a minute amount of cholesterol. It is needed to maintain cell membranes, especially in nerve tissue. It also is an important chemical in the body's manufacture of bile (a substance that is instrumental in our digestion of fats). And cholesterol is a necessity if the body is to make steroid and sex hormones. When your skin is exposed to the sun, cholesterol and other similar compounds are converted into vitamin D; this enables your body to absorb calcium and to maintain your bone structure and teeth, and to carry out other vital functions. In short, if your body were suddenly stripped of all its cholesterol, you would not be able to live. Yet too much available cholesterol in the blood—like too much of all good things—is bad.

Cholesterol is found only in animal products. Egg yolks, liver, and other organ meats are particularly high in cholesterol. Ounce for ounce, most meats, poultry, and fish contain about the same amount of cholesterol—another fact that comes as a great surprise to many people who have been led to believe that only eggs and red meat have cholesterol and that foods such as chicken and fish are either low in cholesterol or free of it. As Table 4 (pages 60–61) shows, foods that vary in the amounts and types of other fats (lipids) they contain may be pretty much equal in cholesterol.

Even though cholesterol is essential for maintaining life, it is not necessary to consume any in the diet. Your body has the capability of making all the cholesterol that it needs. Thus, even very strict vegetarians who shun all animal products, thereby consuming no cholesterol, will not become deficient in it. This is because most of the body's cholesterol is manufactured by the liver; some researchers believe that it is also made in the cells of other organs as well.

Cholesterol is carried through the body via the bloodstream. Since blood is mostly water, and since cholesterol (like other lipids) does not mix with water, it must be attached to another compound—specifically, a protein—in

Table 4. Cholesterol/Fat Content of Foods

FOOD	CHOLESTEROL MG	FATS (gm)		
		SATURATED	MONO-UNSATURATED	POLY-UNSATURATED
1 ounce lean beef	26	0.9	0.8	0.1
1 ounce fatty beef	27	2.2	2.0	0.2
1 ounce veal	28	0.9	0.8	0.1
1 ounce chicken (dark meat)	26	0.8	1.0	0.6
1 ounce chicken/turkey (white meat)	22	0.3	0.3	0.2
1 ounce pork	28	0.9	0.8	0.1
1 ounce beef liver	83	0.1	0	0
1 ounce lean fish	28	0	0.1	0.1
1 ounce fatty fish	25	0.9	1.1	1.1
1 ounce water-packed tuna	11	0	0	0
1 ounce lean lamb	17	0.1	0.2	0.2
1 egg	274	1.7	2.2	0.7

1 tablespoon margarine (1.6/1.9 poly/sat)	2.4	3.3	1.4	0
1 tablespoon corn oil	2.6	1.1	0.6	0
1 tablespoon safflower oil	3.3	0.6	0.4	0
1 tablespoon veg. oil	2.6	1.0	0.7	0
2 tablespoon avocado	1.3	2.1	0.8	0
1 tablespoon butter	0.2	1.4	1.9	12
2 ounces 5% fat cheese	0.1	1.0	1.6	20
2 ounces cheddar	0.5	6.0	12.0	56
1 cup whole milk	0.1	2.4	4.8	34
1 cup 2% milk	0.1	2.0	2.4	22
1 cup skim milk	0	0.1	0.3	4
1 cup 1% yogurt	0.1	1.0	2.3	14
1 cup ice cream	0.3	9.6	16.8	56

order to travel in the blood. The combination is called a lipoprotein. Cholesterol can be categorized according to the type of lipoprotein in which it is combined, as will be explained later in the chapter.

WHEN IS CHOLESTEROL A PROBLEM?

Cholesterol becomes a risk factor only when too much of it circulates in the bloodstream. Your doctor refers to this as "blood cholesterol." As indicated above, until recently there has been no clear agreement as to what constitutes high blood cholesterol. Then in 1987, the National Cholesterol Education Program was established by the National Heart, Lung and Blood Institute to formulate a consensus concerning guidelines for all persons over the age of twenty. They defined the various blood cholesterol levels as follows:

Blood cholesterol level	Category
Less than 200 mg/dl	Desirable blood cholesterol
200 to 239 mg/dl	Borderline-high blood cholesterol
240 mg/dl and above	High blood cholesterol

Cholesterol is also classified according to the type of lipoprotein in which it is incorporated. The most abundant are the low density lipoproteins, or LDL cholesterol. This is often called the "bad" cholesterol because it is the type that is implicated in the development of atherosclerosis. Another type, very low density lipoproteins or VLDL, incorporate mostly triglycerides—the most abundant of the lipids. Although much is known about triglycerides chemically and metabolically, their precise role in heart disease is not as well documented as that of cholesterol. However, a very high level of triglycerides may also be a major risk factor.

In contrast, high density lipoproteins (or the HDL cholesterol) serve to clear cholesterol out of the artery walls, and thus are considered the "good" or beneficial cholesterol. The higher your level of HDL cholesterol compared to LDL cholesterol, the better is your risk. If your total cholesterol is below 200 milligrams per decaliter, it's reasonably safe to assume that your LDL/HDL ratio is fine. If your total cholesterol is above 200 mg/dl, however, the National Cholesterol Education Program recommends that you have further testing, both to confirm the total level and also to determine how much of the cholesterol is HDL or LDL. An LDL level of 130 mg/dl or less is considered desirable. If you are a middle-aged man and your LDL cholesterol is 160 mg/dl or higher, your risk of early death from a heart attack is double that of your peers whose LDL cholesterol levels are in the desirable range. And the higher your LDL cholesterol, the higher your risk. The Framingham Heart Study and a number of other epidemiological studies have found that the risk of a heart attack for a middle-aged man whose LDL cholesterol is 190 mg/dl or higher is four to five times greater than for men whose LDL cholesterol is 130 mg/dl or lower. Figures 2 and 3 (pages 64–65) summarize the National Cholesterol Education Program's recommendations for testing and follow-up based on various blood cholesterol levels.

Figure 2. Initial Evaluation and Classification Based on Total Cholesterol

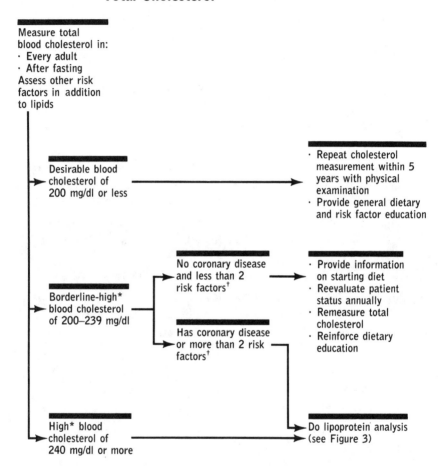

*Must be confirmed by second test
†Including male sex
SOURCE: National Cholesterol Education Program, U.S. Department of Health and Human Services, 1988.

Figure 3. Follow-up Evaluation and Action Based on LDL-cholesterol

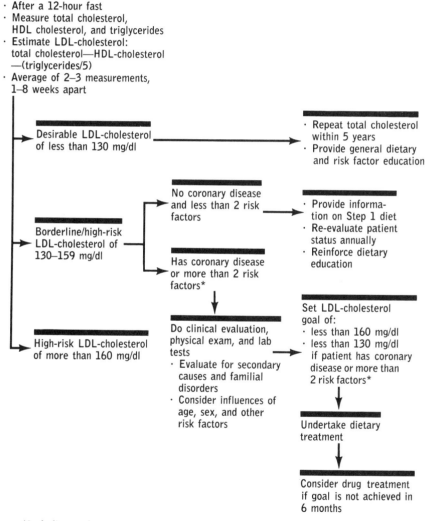

Do lipoprotein analysis
· After a 12-hour fast
· Measure total cholesterol,
  HDL cholesterol, and triglycerides
· Estimate LDL-cholesterol:
  total cholesterol—HDL-cholesterol
  —(triglycerides/5)
· Average of 2–3 measurements,
  1–8 weeks apart

Desirable LDL-cholesterol of less than 130 mg/dl

· Repeat total cholesterol within 5 years
· Provide general dietary and risk factor education

Borderline/high-risk LDL-cholesterol of 130–159 mg/dl

No coronary disease and less than 2 risk factors

· Provide information on Step 1 diet
· Re-evaluate patient status annually
· Reinforce dietary education

Has coronary disease or more than 2 risk factors*

High-risk LDL-cholesterol of more than 160 mg/dl

Do clinical evaluation, physical exam, and lab tests
· Evaluate for secondary causes and familial disorders
· Consider influences of age, sex, and other risk factors

Set LDL-cholesterol goal of:
· less than 160 mg/dl
· less than 130 mg/dl if patient has coronary disease or more than 2 risk factors*

Undertake dietary treatment

Consider drug treatment if goal is not achieved in 6 months

*Including male sex
SOURCE: National Cholesterol Education Program, U.S. Department of Health and Human Services, 1988.

WHAT CAUSES HIGH BLOOD CHOLESTEROL?

Many factors participate in producing a high blood cholesterol, but a combination of genetic predisposition and diet appears to be the most significant. On the average, your body uses about 1,000 milligrams of cholesterol each day for normal functions. About two-thirds of this is made (or synthesized) by the liver and the remainder comes from the diet. Normally, if you eat more cholesterol than you need, your liver will simply cut back on the amount it makes and more will be excreted from the body. However, there are limits to how much the liver will cut back its normal production. Studies have found that people whose diets are very high in cholesterol tend to have high blood cholesterol levels.

Consumption of certain kinds of fats in the foods we eat may be even more important than dietary cholesterol in raising the blood level. For example, saturated fats—the kind that are hard at room temperature, or that are found in tropical oils—tend to raise blood cholesterol levels perhaps even more than foods higher in cholesterol content. In contrast, polyunsaturated and monounsaturated fats—the kinds that are in most vegetable oils, poultry, and fish—tend to lower blood cholesterol.

The kinds of fat that are mostly polyunsaturated include:

Corn oil	Safflower oil
Cottonseed oil	Soybean oil
Fish	Sunflower oil
Margarine	
(especially corn or soft)	

The mostly monounsaturated fats are included in:

Avocado	Olives and olive oil
Cashews	Peanuts and peanut oil

Peanut butter
Poultry   Vegetable shortening
The mostly saturated include:
Butter   Egg yolk
Cheese   Lard
Chocolate   Meat
Coconut and coconut oil   Palm oil

For reasons that are still not fully understood, some people will make too much cholesterol in their liver even if their diet contains moderate or low amounts of cholesterol and fats. Some of these people will turn out to have an inherited disorder called familial hypercholesterolemia. These people comprise a minority of those with high blood cholesterol levels; but they have a more serious form of the disease. From a very early age, they have very high levels of blood cholesterol; and if the disease is not diagnosed and treated, most will have heart attacks or die suddenly at an early age—often in their twenties or thirties.

More commonly, a person with elevated cholesterol levels will have an inherited predisposition to produce or retain a more moderate excess of cholesterol. This hereditable trait, however, does not seem to be as severe a disease as familial hypercholesterolemia. Fortunately, these people do fine just as long as they consume a prudent diet—one that is low in cholesterol and fat (especially saturated fats), and provides enough calories to maintain a desirable weight. In fact, prudent is the term used by the American Heart Association in its dietary recommendations for all of us, those with normal as well as with elevated cholesterol levels.

Although genetics and diet may be the most important factors in determining the blood cholesterol level, they are by no means the only ones. Other factors that also affect cholesterol include:

Obesity and body fat distribution. People who are overweight tend to have high cholesterol levels. In addition, their LDL cholesterol tends to be high and their HDL cholesterol low. Where fat is stored in our body also seems to be important. Excess weight in men and women after menopause tends to be centered in the abdominal area—the so-called pot belly. Recent studies indicate that this fat distribution appears to be associated with elevated blood cholesterol levels more than fat that is stored elsewhere in the body. One explanation is that abdominal fat seems to be more metabolically active. The good news is that with weight reduction, cholesterol levels seem to fall substantially; and the LDL/HDL ratio also improves.

Age. As we get older, our blood cholesterol levels tend to rise somewhat. Thus, what may be a more acceptable level for persons in their fifties or sixties may be much too high for a young adult.

Gender. Men tend to have higher levels of LDL cholesterol than premenopausal women; this is believed to be one reason why men have more heart attacks than premenopausal women. After menopause, however, the LDL cholesterol rises in women; their incidence of heart attacks also rises, so that eventually there is no difference between the two sexes. It is of interest that estrogen replacement therapy may prevent this rise in cholesterol, and some studies have suggested that older women who take estrogen may have a reduced risk of heart attacks. (It should be noted, however, that there may be other hazards involved in taking hormones, including an increased risk of some types of cancer.)

Cigarette smoking. Smokers tend to have low levels of the protective HDL cholesterol, which rise again when they stop smoking. In addition, smoking itself is an in-dependent risk factor for heart disease, and smokers who have high cholesterol have a much greater incidence of heart attacks than do nonsmokers with similarly elevated cholesterol levels.

Diabetes mellitus.   People with diabetes also tend to have high levels of blood cholesterol. This may be related, in part, to the tendency of people with adult onset (Type II) diabetes to be overweight. However, even diabetic patients with normal weight often have high cholesterol levels, and diabetic patients even with normal cholesterol levels have an increased risk for heart attacks and strokes. The major con-cern for these patients is control of body weight, blood sugar, and blood cholesterol levels. This is best assured by regular checkups regarding these factors (and for elevated blood pressure) for any individual with a family history of diabetes.

Drugs.   Some medications raise cholesterol or alter the LDL/HDL ratio. Of particular concern are recent findings that young athletes who use anabolic steroids for muscle building have very low levels of the protective HDL cholesterol. Moreover, any patient with a family history of elevated cholesterol levels or diabetes should have periodic checks of cholesterol when receiving certain therapeutic agents including diuretics, steroids, and even beta-adrenergic receptor blocking agents used to treat other heart conditions.

Miscellaneous factors.   Stress has been linked to a rise in blood cholesterol, but the mechanisms for this remain unresolved. Studies also have found that excessive coffee consumption—more than seven or eight cups a day—may also elevate blood cholesterol levels.

HOW DO YOU LOWER ELEVATED BLOOD CHOLESTEROL?

Most people can reduce their blood cholesterol level—and consequently their risk of a heart attack—by modifying their diet. As stressed by the National Cholesterol Education Program, "This doesn't mean giving up all the foods you love. Instead, you can learn to prepare foods differently and eat certain foods less often and in smaller amounts."

Throughout this book, we have emphasized moderation and modification as the keys to reducing risk factors, rather than absolute restriction and rigidity. This is certainly true for lowering high blood cholesterol. Table 5 (pages 72–74) outlines the dietary recommendations from the National Cholesterol Education Program. The program's four major recommendations are:

Eat less fat. Fats should contribute no more than 30 percent of your total daily calories.

Eat less saturated fat. When it comes to raising blood cholesterol levels, some fats are more detrimental than others. In fact, saturated fats—especially those in milk, butter, cheese, ice cream, and other whole milk products; meats, such as beef, pork, liver, sweetbreads; and tropical plant or tree oils—raise blood cholesterol more than any other component of your diet. The American Heart Association recommends that less than 10 percent of your total calories come from saturated fats. This constitutes about half the amount of saturated fats now consumed in the average diet.

Eat less cholesterol. As noted earlier, dietary cholesterol can raise blood levels. Cholesterol is found only in animal food products—egg yolks and organs meats are our richest sources. The National Cholesterol Education Program recommends that you eat no more than three egg yolks a week, and that you try to limit your total cholesterol intake to less than 300 milligrams a day. Cutting back on meat, poultry, fish, and dairy products can help achieve this goal.

Lose excess weight. As already indicated, overweight people often have high blood cholesterol, and getting rid of excess pounds usually lowers the cholesterol—often to normal levels. Here again, cutting back on animal fats will help achieve your goal. Remember that 1 gram of fat contains 9 calories, compared to 4 calories in 1 gram of carbohydrates or 1 gram of protein. Therefore, a plate of pasta with tomato sauce can be as tasty and filling as a steak, but with none of the cholesterol and far fewer calories. (See Chapter 7 for more detailed tips on losing weight.)

Table 5. Recommended Diet Modifications to Lower Blood Cholesterol

	Choose	Decrease
Fish, Chicken, Turkey, and Lean Meats	Fish, poultry without skin, lean cuts of beef, lamb, pork or veal, shellfish	Fatty cuts of beef, lamb, pork; spare ribs, organ meats, regular cold cuts, sausage, hot dogs, bacon, sardines, roe
Skim and Low-Fat Milk, Cheese, Yogurt, and Dairy Substitutes	Skim or 1% fat milk (liquid, powdered, evaporated), buttermilk	Whole milk (4% fat): regular, evaporated, condensed; cream, half-and-half, 2% milk, imitation milk products, most nondairy creamers, whipped toppings
	Nonfat (0% fat) or low-fat yogurt	Whole-milk yogurt
	Low-fat cottage cheese (1% or 2% fat)	Whole-milk cottage cheese (4% fat)
	Low-fat cheeses, farmer, or pot cheese (all of these should be labeled no more than 2–6 g fat/ounce)	All natural cheeses (e.g., blue, roquefort, camembert, cheddar, Swiss)
		Low-fat or "light" cream cheese, low-fat or "light" sour cream

	Choose	**Decrease**
		Cream cheeses, sour cream
	Sherbet	Ice cream
Eggs	Egg whites (2 whites = 1 whole egg in recipes), cholesterol-free egg substitutes	Egg yolks
Fruits and Vegetables	Fresh, frozen, canned, or dried fruits and vegetables	Vegetables prepared in butter, cream, or other sauces
Breads and Cereals	Homemade baked goods using unsaturated oils sparingly, angel food cake, low-fat crackers, low-fat cookies Rice, pasta Whole-grain breads and cereals (oatmeal, whole wheat, rye, bran, multigrain, etc.)	Commercial baked goods: pies, cakes, doughnuts, croissants, pastries, muffins, biscuits, high-fat crackers, high-fat cookies Egg noodles Breads in which eggs are major ingredient
Fats and Oils	Baking cocoa Unsaturated vegetable oils; corn, olive, rapeseed (canola oil), safflower, sesame, soybean, sunflower	Chocolate Butter, coconut oil, palm oil, palm kernel oil, lard, bacon fat

Choose	Decrease
Margarine or shortening made from one of the unsaturated oils listed above	
Diet margarine	Dressings made
Mayonnaise, salad dressings made with unsaturated oils listed above	with egg yolks
Low-fat dressings	
Seeds and nuts	Coconut

SOURCE: National Cholesterol Education Program, 1988, National Heart, Lung and Blood Institute.

OTHER CHOLESTEROL-LOWERING STRATEGIES

While some foods raise blood cholesterol, there are others that can help lower it. Perhaps the most notable cholesterol-lowering foods are those that are high in soluble fiber. Of these, oat bran recently has garnered the most publicity, and studies have found that a diet that includes 10 to 12 grams of oat bran will reduce blood cholesterol. To get this much oat bran, however, you would have to eat two large bowls of oatmeal and a medium-size oat bran muffin. Many people find that this much bran will produce bloating, intestinal gas, and diarrhea. To overcome that problem, you can cut back on the oat bran a bit and substitute foods that are high in other soluble fibers such as pectin (found in apples and berries), guar (used as a filler in many foods), or the fiber in dried peas, beans, lentils, and other legumes. Other grains, including rice, are under study at present and may turn out to have similarly beneficial or even better effects.

Fish oils, particularly those high in omega-3 fatty acids, also have been widely promoted in recent years for their cholesterol-lowering value. While there is sound epidemiological evidence showing that people who eat fish two or three times a week have a reduced incidence of heart attacks, the same cannot be said for taking fish oil extracts. According to Dr. Virgil Brown, head of the National Cholesterol Education Program's diet subcommittee, fish oil extracts "do not lower LDL cholesterol or specifically raise HDL cholesterol, and are, therefore, not recommended as treatment of an elevated cholesterol." He further warns that fish oil extracts alter the blood's clotting ability, and may cause bleeding problems, especially if you already are taking low-dose aspirin or other blood thinners to prevent a heart attack. This is particularly important for patients with hypertension since they are particularly predisposed to hemorrhagic strokes; the bleeding could then be all the more life-threatening.

There are many easy ways to modify your present diet to reduce your cholesterol without resorting to fads of dietary supplements. Here are some specific tips from the National Cholesterol Education Program:

Master the fine art of food substitution. Almost every high-fat, high-cholesterol food has a low-fat, low-cholesterol counterpart—all you have to do is look and experiment a bit. For example, if you love ice cream (and who doesn't?), try one of the low-fat varieties (check the label, however, since some are made with tropical oils). Better still, switch to a low-fat ice milk, sherbet, yogurt, or nonfat sorbet. Commerical pastries and other baked goods often are made with tropical oils; make your own or switch to things like ginger snaps or angel food cake. Use skim or 1 percent fat milk instead of whole milk; look for nonfat yogurt and skim or part-skim milk cheeses.

Trim meats and discard the fat. Buy lean cuts to begin with, then trim or scrape off any visible fat. Remove the skin from poultry and trim off the fat. Avoid self-basting turkeys, which have injected fats, often butter or tropical oils.

Use low-fat seasonings and sauces. Look for low-fat mayonnaise and spreads or use low-fat alternatives like mustard. Season vegetables with spices and herbs instead of butter, cheese, and cream sauces. Top a baked potato with yogurt and fresh chives or dill instead of butter, sour cream, or cheese.

Use low-fat cooking methods. Broil, grill, roast, or steam foods instead of frying. If you do fry, use a nonstick pan and pan spray instead of butter or fat. Try poaching foods in broth or wine; cook stews and soups ahead of time, chill, then skim off the hardened fat before reheating and serving. Discard pan dripplings or at least skim off all the fat before using. Don't put potatoes or other vegetables in your roast—vegetables cooked this way tend to soak up the fat. Avoid coating mixes; commercial ones are loaded with fats, including tropical oils, and even homemade ones will soak up all the fat in a pan.

Experiment with reducing the fat in recipes. You usually can cut the fat in recipes by one-third to even one-half without changing the texture or flavor. Use margarine or oil instead of butter, lard, and vegetable shortening (which is usually made with tropical oils). Yogurt, or cheese made by straining yogurt, can be used instead of sour cream or cream cheese in most recipes. If a recipe calls for eggs, discard half of the yolks or, better still, discard all the yolks and substitute 2 egg whites and 2 teaspoons of vegetable oil for each egg. (If you can't bear to throw away the yolks, give them to your

cat or dog—their bodies metabolize cholesterol and fats differently from humans, and an occasional egg yolk is good for
their skin and fur.)
   **Cut portion sizes of high-fat or high-cholesterol
foods.** Use meats and cheese as components of another
recipe instead of a separate main course. For example, instead
of serving a whole steak, cut a few ounces into strips and mix
it with stir-fried vegetables. Use a sprinkling of parmesan
instead of a thick layer of cheese on pizza or pasta. Increase
the vegetables and cut back on meat in stews. Use yogurt or
low-fat cottage cheese instead of ricotta in cheese cake; substitute low-fat cottage cheese and vegetables for meat and
cheese in lasagna and other pasta dishes.
   Check labels when shopping. You may be surprised
to find that those so-called cholesterol-lowering oat bran
muffins, cereals, and cookies also contain cholesterol-raising
tropical oils. Or that cholesterol-free nondairy coffee cream-
ers are mostly cholesterol-raising palm or coconut oils. Even
some egg substitutes are made with tropical oils. (See Table
6, pages 78–83, for a guide to shopping.)

WHEN DIET ALONE IS NOT ENOUGH

Some people simply cannot lower their blood cholesterol
enough through dietary measures alone. The National
Cholesterol Education Program recommends that anyone
whose blood cholesterol level is in the borderline-high or
high category should be given specific dietary counseling. If
six months of a conscientious trial of dietary changes does
not bring down the total cholesterol and LDL cholesterol to a
predetermined level (preferably an LDL cholesterol of 130
mg/dl or lower), then cholesterol-lowering drugs may be
prescribed. A number of different ones are now available,

Table 6. A Guide to Choosing Low-Fat, Low-Cholesterol Foods

Variety is the spice of life. Choose foods every day from each of the following food groups. Choose different foods from within groups, especially foods low in saturated fat and cholesterol (the Choose column). As a guide, the recommended daily number of servings for adults is listed for each food group. But you'll have to decide on the number of servings you need to lose or maintain your weight. If you need help, ask a dietitian or your doctor.

	Choose	Go Easy On	Decrease
Meat, Poultry, Fish, and Shellfish (up to 6 ounces a day)	*Lean cuts* of meat with fat trimmed, like: ■ beef—round, sirloin, chuck, loin ■ lamb—leg, arm, loin, rib ■ pork—tenderloin, leg (fresh), shoulder (arm or picnic) ■ veal—all trimmed cuts except ground Poultry without skin Fish, shellfish		"Prime" grade *Fatty cuts* of meat like: ■ beef—corned beef brisket, regular ground, short ribs ■ pork—spareribs, blade roll Goose, domestic duck Organ meats, like liver, kidney, sweetbread, brain Sausage, bacon Regular luncheon meats Frankfurters Caviar, roe

Dairy Products (2 servings a day; 3 servings for women who are pregnant or breast-feeding)	Skim milk, 1% milk, low-fat buttermilk, low-fat evaporated or nonfat milk Low-fat yogurt Low-fat soft cheeses, like cottage, farmer, pot Cheeses labeled no more than 2 to 6 grams of fat an ounce	2% milk Yogurt Part-skim ricotta Part-skim or imitation hard cheeses, like part-skim mozzarella "Light" cream cheese "Light" sour cream	Whole milk like regular, evaporated, condensed Cream, half-and-half, most nondairy creamers and products, real or nondairy whipped cream Cream cheese Sour cream Custard-style yogurt Whole-milk ricotta High-fat cheeses, like neufchatel, brie, Swiss, American, mozzarella, feta, cheddar, muenster
Eggs (no more than 3 egg yolks a week)	Egg whites Cholesterol-free egg substitutes		Egg yolks

	Choose	Go Easy On	Decrease
Fats and Oils (up to 6 to 8 teaspoons a day)	Unsaturated vegetable oils: corn, olive, peanut, rapeseed (canola oil), safflower, sesame, soybean; Margarine or shortening made with unsaturated fats listed above: liquid, tub, stick, diet mayonnaise, salad dressings made with unsaturated fats listed above; Low-fat dressings	Nuts and seeds; Avocados and olives	Butter, coconut oil, palm kernel oil, palm oil, lard, bacon fat; Margarine or shortening made with saturated fats listed above; Dressings made with egg yolk
Breads, Cereals, Pasta, Rice, Dried Peas and Beans (6 to 11 servings a day)	Breads, like white, whole-wheat, pumpernickel, and rye breads; pita; bagels; English	Store-bought pancakes, waffles, biscuits, muffins, cornbread	Croissants, butter rolls, sweet rolls, Danish pastry, doughnuts; Most snack crackers, like cheese crackers,

muffins; sandwich buns; dinner rolls; rice cakes

Low-fat crackers, like matzo, bread sticks, rye krisp, saltines, zwieback

Hot cereals, most cold dry cereals

Pasta, like plain noodles, spaghetti, macaroni

Any grain rice

Dried peas and beans, like split peas, black-eyed peas, chick peas, kidney beans, navy beans, lentils, soybeans, soybean curd (tofu)

butter crackers, those made with saturated fats

Granola-type cereals made with saturated fats

Pasta and rice prepared with cream, butter, or cheese sauces; egg noodles

	Choose	Go Easy On	Decrease
Fruits and Vegetables (2 to 4 servings of fruit and 3 to 5 servings of vegetables a day)	Fresh, frozen, canned, or dried fruits and vegetables		Vegetables prepared in butter, cream, or sauce
Sweets and Snacks (avoid too many sweets)	Low-fat frozen desserts, like sherbet, sorbet, Italian ice, frozen yogurt, popsicles Low-fat cakes, like angel food cake Low-fat cookies, like fig bars, gingersnaps Low-fat candy, like jelly beans, hard candy Low-fat snacks, like plain popcorn, pretzels Nonfat beverages, like carbonated drinks, juices, tea, coffee	Frozen desserts, like ice milk Homemade cakes, cookies, and pies using unsaturated oils sparingly Fruit crisps and cobblers Potato and corn chips prepared with unsaturated vegetable oil	High-fat frozen desserts, like ice cream, frozen tofu High-fat cakes, like most store-bought, pound, and frosted cakes Store-bought pies Most store-bought cookies Most candy, like chocolate bars Potato and corn chips prepared with saturated fat Buttered popcorn High-fat beverages, like frappes, milkshakes, floats, and eggnogs

Label Ingredients

To avoid too much fat or saturated fat, go easy on products that list any fat or oil first or that list many fat and oil ingredients. The following lists name unsaturated fat ingredients and saturated fat or high-cholesterol ingredients that do or do not fit well in a cholesterol-lowering diet.

Unsaturated Fat Ingredients

Carob, cocoa
Oils, like corn, cottonseed, olive, safflower, sesame, soybean, or sunflower
Nonfat dry milk, nonfat dry milk solids, skim milk

Saturated Fat or High Cholesterol Ingredients

Chocolate
Animal fat, like bacon, beef, ham, lamb, meat, pork, chicken or turkey fats, butter, lard
Coconut, coconut oil, palm kernel or palm oil
Cream
Egg and egg-yolk solids
Hardened fat or oil
Hydrogenated vegetable oil
Shortening or vegetable shortening
Unspecified vegetable oil (could be coconut, palm kernel, or palm oil)

Prepared by the National Cholesterol Education Program, National Heart, Lung and Blood Institute which are described and summarized in Table 7 (pages 86–87). And more effective ones are in the wings at present. Specific cholesterol lowering drugs include:

Bile acid sequestrants. This class of drugs, which includes cholestyramine and colestipol, are among the first-choice drugs recommended by the National Cholesterol Education Program. They effectively lower LDL cholesterol, and their long-term safety has been established by a number of scientific studies. A large-scale study carried out at several medical centers also demonstrated that they reduce the incidence of heart attacks.

These drugs work by binding to bile acids in the intestinal tract. This prevents the return of the bile acids to the liver, and to replace them, the liver converts more cholesterol into new bile acids. In effect, this reduces the amount of LDL cholesterol circulating in the blood.

Both cholestyramine and colestipol come in powder form, which can be dissolved in water or fruit juice and consumed with meals. In the past, many patients complained of the gritty taste, but this problem has been minimized with new formulations. The drugs are not absorbed into the bloodstream, so their side effects are limited to the gastrointestinal tract; the most common are bloating, a feeling of fullness, flatulence, nausea, and constipation. They generally are not recommended for patients with chronic constipation, although they also may be taken in conjunction with a laxative.

Although the drugs are not absorbed themselves, they may interfere with the body's absorption of fat-soluble vitamins (A, D. E, and K), folic acid, and a number of medications, including digitoxin (a heart medication), thyroid hormone replacement, warfarin (a blood-thinning drug), thiazide diuretics, and beta blockers. Your doctor should know of any medication you are taking before prescribing these (or any other medications), to prevent adverse interactions.

Nicotinic acid. This is a form of niacin, one of the B vitamins. When taken in very large doses, nicotinic acid acts like a drug, lowering LDL cholesterol and triglycerides and raising HDL cholesterol. It is the other first-choice medication recommended by the National Cholesterol Education Program. It works by lowering the liver's production of VLDL cholesterol, which in turn reduces the manufacture of LDL cholesterol.

Side effects are a major problem with high-dose nicotinic acid, but these usually can be controlled by adjusting the dosage. Itching and hot flushes are the most common side effects. The flushing may be controlled or minimized by taking the nicotinic acid at meals, by gradually building up the dosage, by using a time-release form of the drug, or by taking it with aspirin or a nonsteroidal anti-inflammatory drug (ibuprofen or other similar drugs commonly used to treat arthritis and pain). Very high doses carry a risk of liver abnormalities, increased levels of uric acid (which can lead to attacks of gout), and high blood sugar. Although these side effects are relatively uncommon, patients on nicotinic acid should have periodic blood tests to make sure they are not occurring.

It should be noted that nicotinamide, an alternative form of niacin, does not have the same cholesterol-lowering effects as nicotinic acid. Although it has been promoted as an alternative to nicotinic acid that does not cause flushing, it should not be used as a substitute to lower cholesterol.

Liver enzyme (HMG CoA reductase) inhibitors. These are the newest cholesterol-lowering drugs, with the highly publicized lovastatin being the only one approved for use in the United States. They work through

Table 7. Major Drugs to Lower Cholesterol for Consideration

Drugs	Reduce Coronary Disease Risk	Long-Term Safety	Maintaining Adherence	Lowering of LDL-cholesterol	Special Precaution
Cholestyramine Colestipol	Yes	Yes	Requires considerable education	15–30%	Can alter absorption of other drugs; can increase triglyceride levels and should not be used in patients with hypertriglyceridemia
Nicotinic acid	Yes	Yes	Requires considerable education	15–30%	Test for hyperuricemia, hyperglycemia, and liver function abnormalities.

Lovastatin	Not proven	Not established	Relatively easy	25–45%	Monitor for liver function abnormalities and possible lens opacities
Probucol	Not proven	Not established	Relatively easy	10–15%	Lowers HDL-cholesterol (significance has not been established); may alter heart's electrical activity as indicated by changes in the QT interval on an ECG.

SOURCE: National Cholesterol Education Program, National Heart, Lung and Blood Institute.

the liver by inhibiting the enzyme (HMG CoA reductase) responsible for synthesis of cholesterol. Although lovastatin may lower LDL cholesterol by 25 to 40 percent, it is not among the first-choice drugs recommended by the National Cholesterol Education Program. Its long-term safety has not been established and it also is more costly than the bile acid sequestrants and nicotinic acid.

The most common side effects to date have been changes in bowel function, headaches, nausea, fatigue, insomnia, skin rashes, and changes in liver function. These side effects have been reported in less than 5 percent of patients, but more study is needed to establish their long-term safety.

Miscellaneous other drugs. Probucol has been shown to reduce LDL cholesterol by about 8 to 15 percent, but this benefit is offset by an even larger (up to 25 percent) reduction in HDL cholesterol. It is sometimes used to treat patients who cannot tolerate other cholesterol-lowering drugs, but the National Cholesterol Education Program does not recommend its routine use. Side effects include diarrhea, flatulence, abdominal cramps, and nausea, but these occur in less than 5 percent of patients.

Gemfibrozil and clofibrate, both medications in a class called fibric acid derivatives, are used primarily to lower triglycerides. They also lower LDL cholesterol and raise HDL cholesterol. Both drugs are generally well tolerated, but they may cause gastrointestinal upsets and have adverse effects on the blood. The long-term safety of these drugs has not been established, although studies indicate that clofibrate may cause long-term toxicity.

6 OVERCOMING "FAT" GENES

"I was born to be fat and there's nothing I can do about it."
Sally Arthur, the patient who made this simple declaration,
had recently suffered a minor heart attack. Although she was
lucky in that she incurred little damage to her heart, it was
imperative that she lose weight to reduce her risk of another
heart attack. Sally was firmly convinced that she had inherited her weight problem, and that no matter what she did,
she was destined to be fat. Recent research seems to confirm
that there is, indeed, a genetic or inherited tendency to gain
weight. But it certainly is not true that there is nothing a
person with such a genetic tendency can do to keep from
being overweight.

It's no secret that as Americans, we are obsessed with
weight—and with some justification. The recent surgeon
general's report on nutrition and health notes that some 34
million American adults are obese, making it the "most
prevalent diet-related problem in the United States."

According to this report: "As the diseases of nutritional deficiency have diminished, they have been replaced by diseases of dietary excess and imbalance—problems that now rank among the leading causes of illness and death in the United States."

Indeed, of the ten leading causes of death in this country, four are associated with diet and excess weight—heart disease, stroke, diabetes mellitus, and some types of cancer. Obesity is closely linked to several major cardiovascular risk factors. For example, people who are overweight tend to have high levels of blood cholesterol. Excessive weight also promotes high blood pressure and adult-onset diabetes.

Obesity is also associated with a number of other conditions that may not be life-threatening, but are still costly and disabling. These include degenerative arthritis, gout, gallbladder disease, and several digestive system disorders.

Like millions of fellow overweight Americans, even before her heart attack Sally Arthur, a secretary in a law firm, had approached her weight problem by dieting. "I've tried them all," she said. "Scarsdale, Atkins, Cambridge, Beverly Hills, the Diamonds . . . just name it and I've been on it. Do they work? Just look at me! Sure, I've lost weight on every one of them, but it just doesn't stay off."

CALORIES AND WEIGHT CONTROL

It's well known that fad or crash diets simply do not work. While these diets have different trappings, they also have two important things in common: they promise fast, painless weight loss and they use some sort of gimmick to reduce caloric intake. People following these various dietary regimens do lose weight, simply because they are taking in less calories than they burn up, forcing the body to turn to its fat (and lean tissue as well) in order to meet its energy needs.

Their fatal flaw, however, is that they do not attack the real underlying problem for most obese individuals—faulty eating habits. Even if a person is genetically predisposed to gain weight, it's eating more than the body needs that puts on the extra pounds. The basic premise of most weight-reduction diets is to deny yourself food for a certain period of time, shed the desired number of pounds, and then reward yourself by going off the diet. To most people, this means resuming former eating habits, which caused the overweight in the first place. Before long, the excess fat is back, often with a few more pounds for good measure. So it's back on the diet, and the scenario is played out again—and again and again.

Unfortunately, this all-too-common "yo-yo" approach to weight control is self-defeating for several reasons. One has to do with effects on the body's overall metabolism. Your body needs a certain amount of fuel (energy or calories) just to carry out its basic vital functions such as breathing, circulation, digestion, and even thinking. For example, when you are sleeping, you are burning up a certain number of calories. This basic energy requirement is referred to as basal metabolism. In addition, your body requires calories to carry out day-to-day activities. How many extra calories you need in addition to energy required to support basal metabolism depends upon the extent of your physical activity. Obviously, you will need more calories if you are a professional dancer or athlete than if you spend most of your waking hours sitting at a desk or in other sedentary pursuits. (Table 8, pages 92–94, lists the caloric requirements for various physical activities.)

Your total calorie needs can be calculated by adding those needed to maintain basal metabolism to the amount you burn in various activities. (See Table 9, pages 94–95, for a simple formula to calculate your average caloric needs.) When you take in more calories than you expend, the excess is converted into adipose tissue and stored as body fat. When you eat fewer calories than you need, the body can turn to this stored fat, converting it back into a form of energy it can use for various metabolic activities. In simple terms, then, you gain weight (store fat) when you take in more calories than you burn up. And you lose weight when you burn up more calories than you take in.

Easy as this sounds, however, the fact is that weight control is a very difficult and complex process that we still do not fully understand. For example, we do not know why some people get fat while others who seemingly eat the same amount of food (or even more) stay slim. Clearly, heredity, age, and individual metabolic differences all play important roles. But life-style is also important, and even if you have a genetic predisposition to gain weight, the matter is not entirely out of your hands. Through commonsense eating habits and exercise, you can achieve and maintain a desirable weight. You may not be able to turn yourself into a pencil-thin model, but you don't have to be fat, either.

Table 8. Calories Consumed in Various Activities

ACTIVITY	CALORIES PER ½ HOUR
Badminton	175
Basketball	220
Bicycling (5 mph)	105
(6 mph)	135
(8 mph)	165
(10 mph)	195
(11 mph)	225
(13 mph)	330

ACTIVITY	CALORIES PER ½ HOUR
Bowling	135
Canoeing (2 ½ mph)	115
Dancing, aerobic	270
Dancing, ballroom	190
Gardening	110
Golf (using power cart)	100
Golf (pulling cart)	135
Hill climbing (100 ft. per hour)	245
Horseback riding (trotting)	175
Housework (light)	130
Housework (heavy)	210
Ice skating (10 mph)	200
Jogging (5 mph)	265
Racketball	280
Roller skating	175
Rowboating (2 ½ mph)	150
Running (5 mph)	310
(8 mph)	360
(10 mph)	450
Scull rowing (race)	420
Skiing (10 mph)	300
Skiing, crosscountry	330
Squash and handball	300
Square dancing	175
Swimming (¼ mph)	150
Table tennis	180
Tennis, doubles	185

ACTIVITY	CALORIES PER ½ HOUR
Tennis, singles	220
Volleyball	175
Walking (1 mph)	68
(2 mph)	105
(3 mph)	135
(4 mph)	195
(5 mph)	220
Water skiing	240
Weight training, circuit	370

Adapted from the President's Council on Physical Fitness and Sports, Washington, D.C.

Table 9. Calculating Your Average Daily Caloric Needs

Basal metabolic rate (calories needed to sustain vital processes)

For women:
Your weight times 11
Example: 120 pounds × 11 = 1420 calories

For men:
Your weight times 12
Example: 170 pounds × 12 = 2040 calories

Since your metabolic rate decreases with age, you should subtract 2 percent for each decade over the age of 30.
Example: A 41-year-old woman weighing 120 pounds
120 × 11 = 1420 − (4% of 1420 or 57) = 1363 calories

Example: A 54-year-old woman weighing 170 pounds
170 × 12 = 2040 − (6% of 2040 or 122) = 1918 calories

To find your total daily needs, caloric expenditure of normal activities should be added to calories needed to support your basal metabolism. The following formula takes into account both the basal metabolic rate and various levels of physical activity. This formula is for a healthy 20-year-old; find your total and then subtract 2 percent for each decade over the age of 20.

If you are mostly sedentary, multiply your weight by 14.

Example: A sedentary 41-year-old woman weighing 120 pounds 120 × 14 = 1680 − 4% (or 67) = 1613 calories a day.

If you are moderately active, multiply your weight by 15.

Example: A moderately active 54-year-old man weighing 170 pounds 170 × 15 = 2550 − 6% (or 153) = 2397 calories a day.

If you are very active, multiply your weight by 16.

Example: A very active 41-year-old man weighing 120 pounds 120 × 16 = 1920 − 4% (or 77) = 1843 calories a day.

NOTE: The above figures can be rounded off to the nearest tenth. If you find you are gaining or losing weight when you consume the designated amount of calories, adjust accordingly. Some very active people need 18, 20, or even more calories per pound to maintain their desirable weight.

A COMMONSENSE WEIGHT REDUCTION PLAN

If you're like Sally Arthur, and you must lose weight to save your life, a good starting point is to swear off fad diets forever. The promises of fad diets—"Follow me and you'll lose 20 pounds in two weeks without feeling hungry"—is tempting. But don't yield to the temptation, for this is how you get started on the up-and-down diet rollercoaster. Here's what happens.

By definition, crash diets entail the need to sharply curtail your food intake. Your body reacts by conserving as much energy as possible. After all, your body doesn't know that you're deliberately withholding food instead of starving from famine or a concentration camp situation. In any situation in which the body is deprived of adequate fuel, it reacts by slowing down its bodily processes. And the longer you starve yourself, the more marked the metabolic change. It doesn't take long for your metabolic clock to reset itself, so even when you go off the diet and resume eating "normal" amounts of food, your metabolism may still be set to run on "slow." As a result, your body will not require as much energy to perform the same functions as before. So, if your basal metabolism required 1,200 calories before dieting, it may only burn up 1,000 afterward. In other words, even if you eat only as much as was needed to maintain a desirable weight before, now that your body requires fewer calories, there may still be some calories (in this case, 200 a day) left over to store as fat. In no time, an extra 200 calories a day can add up to unwanted pounds. It takes about 3,500 calories to make a pound of fat; so in a little less than five weeks, 200 calories a day will add up to 2 pounds of fat.

This is one reason that repeat dieters find it increasingly more difficult to lose weight. And once the weight is lost, even less food will be needed to put it right back on.

This does not mean, however, that it's impossible to shed unwanted pounds and keep them off. You can fool your metabolic clock and avoid the yo-yo effect by following a commonsense program that provides for a *gradual* weight reduction—no more than 1 or 2 pounds a week. Moreover, if you increase your exercise at the same time you cut back on your caloric intake, you will speed up your metabolism and burn even more calories. This is in contrast to the slowed-down metabolism that normally occurs when you reduce food intake and do not increase exercise. Thus, the chance of maintaining the gradual weight reduction is enhanced and so are your chances of not regaining weight when you reach your desired level. This kind of gradual weight loss may take longer, but you'll win in the end!

Even though this approach makes perfect sense and is medically sound, many patients tend to be skeptical. "I've heard this so many times," Sally Arthur said, echoing the sentiments of many patients in her predicament. "It just won't work for me. I need to see results when I step on that scale, and I need a diet to follow."

The solution? For Sally, it was working closely with a dietitian to develop an eating program (not a "diet") that she could follow for the rest of her life. And the results were reflected in a steady weight loss of 5 or 6 pounds every month until she reached her goal, which was then maintained because there was no diet to go off—she simply continued eating as she had for the past six months. Such an approach may not pack the glamour of Elizabeth Taylor's dramatic weight loss or Oprah Winfrey's transformation, to cite two highly publicized examples. However, it does work and what's more important, it's a lot safer and more apt to be permanent than the fad diet of the moment.

The following is a step-by-step program that you can use to adopt eating habits that will take off pounds and, at the same time, achieve dietary goals designed to reduce other cardiovascular risk factors.

Analyze your present eating habits. Surprisingly, many people are unaware of unhealthy eating habits. Sally Arthur, for example, insisted that she actually ate very little, and that what she did eat was low in calories, sugar, and fats. Her dietitian explained that the best way to spot and correct faulty eating habits entailed keeping a careful food diary for a few days. "Carry this pocket notebook around with you," she instructed, "and write down everything you eat."

Sally was further instructed to write down the food, portion size, time, and circumstances. "Be sure to record what you eat and drink at time of intake," the dietitian said. "Don't wait until the end of the day. By then, it's almost impossible to remember everything you have eaten during the day." Sally also was cautioned not to forget drinks. "People often assume that liquids don't add calories," her dietitian explained. "In fact, drinks can contribute a large number of calories and for many people, make up the difference between being overweight versus normal weight." (See Figure 4 below for a model food diary.)

Figure 4. Personal Food Diary

Make up diary sheets based on the following for at least 5 days. Carry your food diary with you and fill it in each time you eat or drink. Use a pocket calorie counter to calculate the approximate number of calories. Share it with your dietitian or physician to pinpoint areas that need changing and to develop a more healthful eating program.

Personal Food Diary of: _____

Date: _____

Time	Place and Circumstances	Food/Amount	Calories
Example:			
7:30 a.m.	Breakfast at home	1 cup cereal	110
"	"	½ cup skim milk	45
"	"	½ grapefruit	40
"	"	coffee/milk	20
11 a.m.	Snack	English muffin	140
"	"	margarine	30
"	"	jam	20
"	"	cola	150

Total Calories Consumed During Day _____

After a week, Sally returned to the dietitian with her food
diary. (See Figure 5 below.) It was fairly easy to spot Sally's
problem areas. She tended to skip breakfast. "I don't feel
hungry in the mornings, so I figure that's a good time to save
on calories," she explained. "A couple of cups of coffee are all
I need to get me going."

Figure 5.

Personal Food Diary of: *Sally Arthur*

Date: *Tuesday, June 4*

Time	Place and Circumstances	Food/Amount	Calories
7 a.m.	*Home/getting ready for work*	*2 c. coffee w/milk*	*40*
		& sugar	*30*
10:30 a.m.	*Morning break*	*12-ounce cola*	*140*
"	"	*Cheese Danish*	*350*
1 p.m.	*Lunch break*	*12-oz. cola*	*140*
"	"	*Granola bar*	*120*
3 p.m.	*Afternoon break*	*Peanuts, 2 ½ oz.*	*570*
"	"	*12-oz. cola*	*140*
5:30 p.m.	*Fixing supper/hungry*	*2 sl. Am. cheese*	*200*
"	"	*6 Ritz crackers*	*110*
"	"	*Banana (med.)*	*125*
6 p.m.	*Cocktail with husband*	*Manhattan (4 oz.)*	*165*

Time	Place and Circumstances	Food/Amount	Calories
"	"	½ c. goldfish crackers	90
7 p.m.	Dinner with family	½ chicken breast (breaded/fried)	365
"	"	Baked potato	100
"	"	2 T. sour cream	50
"	"	½ cup peas in	60
		cream sauce	120
"	"	1 c. green salad/	50
		2 T. blue cheese dressing	150
		Coffee/mlk/sugar	35
"	"	Gingerbread w/	175
"	"	custard topping	100
8:30 p.m.	Watching TV	3 oz. potato chips	400
"	"	12-oz. beer	150
10 p.m.	Before bed/hungry	½ c. choc. ice cream	135
		cream w/2 oatmeal cookies	120

Total Calories Consumed During Day _____

In midmorning, she'd have another cup of coffee and sometimes a Danish or other pastry to take the edge off her hunger. "That way, I can skip lunch," she reasoned, "so I am actually saving calories." At lunchtime she often went shopping, and would get by on a candy bar and cola.

By midafternoon, Sally would begin to feel very hungry. Hunger is your body's way of telling you it's running low on fuel. As explained earlier, your body has a constant need for a certain amount of energy just to carry on vital processes. When you are awake and moving about, even in a relatively sedentary job, you still need extra energy above your basal metabolic needs. If you skip meals and deny your body a constant supply of food, it sends out hunger signals to let you know that it needs a fresh supply of fuel. If this fuel is not forthcoming from a regular intake of food, your body begins to convert stored energy into fuel.

Many people think that ignoring hunger signals is all a matter of willpower. In reality, it is almost impossible to ignore hunger for a prolonged period. After going without food, your body reacts as if it were in a state of starvation. It will begin to slow down its metabolic rate to conserve as much energy as possible, and at the same time, step up its hunger signals. If food is available, it takes a superhuman effort not to eat.

At her afternoon coffee break, Sally began to make up for all the skimping on food earlier in the day. And from then until bedtime, she actually consumed more calories than she normally would if she were eating a regular breakfast and lunch with one or two small snacks in between.

Draw up a workable eating plan. Sally's dietitian determined that for her age, weight, and level of activity, she needed about 1,800 calories a day to maintain her present weight. She could lose about 1½ pounds a week if she reduced her food intake to about 1,200 calories a day and increased her daily exercise to burn up an extra 200 calories a day. Many weight-loss diets call for 1,000 or fewer calories a day, but Sally's dietitian recommended against a more stringent diet. "You have a long history of crash dieting," she explained. "Our goal is not simply to lose weight, but to get you to your desirable weight and then keep you there for the rest of your life. Remember, it took a lifetime of eating to get you where you are today. You can invest a few months more to get to where you want to be for life."

With careful food choices, Sally could be assured of getting all the nutrients she needed for a healthy diet. By distributing her food intake throughout the entire day, she could avoid feeling hungry.

Using Sally's food diary and a list of her favorite foods, the dietitian worked out a model eating program (see Table 10, pages 104–105). Sally was surprised that it included generous amounts of pasta and other starches—foods she had always thought were fattening. In fact, many experts on weight control recommend that starches make up half or more of your total calories. This also is in keeping with recommendations from the American Heart Association, the American Cancer Society, and the federal government's dietary guidelines for healthy Americans. Specifically, these various guidelines recommend that:

- 60 to 65 percent of calories should come from carbohydrates, with about 10 to 15 percent from simple sugars (preferably the sugars in fruits) and the balance from starches.
- 30 percent or less of total calories should come from fats, with no more than 10 percent from saturated fats.
- About 12 percent should come from protein, either animal protein or a balance of vegetable proteins (i.e., legumes combined with grains) to make whole protein.

Table 10. Model Food Plan for Sally Arthur

Following is an adjusted eating plan based on Sally Arthur's food
diary, showing how her regular meal pattern and food choices
could be modified to give her 1200 calories a day. Portion sizes and
food choices would gradually be increased aftr she reaches her
desired weight.

Time	Place and Circumstances	Food/Amount	Calories
Example:			
7 a.m.	*Breakfast*	*½ grapefruit*	40
"	"	*1 shredded wheat/*	90
		½ c. skim milk	45
		coffee/sugar/milk	35
10:30 a.m.	*Morning break*	*Bran muffin*	105
"	"	*Seltzer*	0
1 p.m.	*Lunch*	*1 c. minestrone soup*	85
"	"	*2 saltines*	25
"	"	*Garden salad/*	50
		1 T. vinaigrette	15
		Tea/lemon	5
3 p.m.	*Afternoon break*	*1 med. apple*	85
"	"	*8 oz. skim milk*	90
5:30	*Fixing supper/hungry*	*2 wheat crackers*	25
6 p.m.	*Cocktail with husband*	*Seltzer*	0
"	"	*Raw vegetables*	20
7 p.m.	*Dinner with family*	*2 oz. roast turkey breast*	
		(no skin)	100
"	"	*Baked potato*	100
"	"	*with chives/pepper*	0

Time	Place and Circumstances	Food/Amount	Calories
Example:			
"	"	½ c. broccoli with lemon	20
		Fresh fruit cup	75
		Coffee w/cinnamon	0
8:30	Watching TV	1 c. chili-flavor popcorn	50
"	"	6 oz. lite beer	50
10 p.m.	Before bed	8 oz. skim milk	90
Total Calories Consumed During Day			1200

Learn to eat in moderation. Any food eaten in excess of what you burn up will be fattening. Ounce for ounce, pasta, potatoes, and other starches tend to be less fattening than most other foods. Remember: 1 gram of carbohydrate or protein contains 4 calories, compared to 9 calories in 1 gram of fat and 7 in 1 gram of alcohol. Starchy foods contain little fat, so they are not as fattening as meats and many high-protein foods, which usually harbor varying amounts of fat.

Even though they may be low in calories, starchy foods tend to be filling, especially if they also contain large amounts of dietary fiber. Fiber does not add appreciable calories to the diet because it is not broken down and digested in the human digestive tract. It absorbs large amounts of water from the stomach and intestines, thereby promoting a feeling of fullness and satiety. Thus, whole-grain cereals and breads, brown rice, and pasta made from whole grains are particularly good choices since they provide good amounts of vitamins and minerals, and their high fiber content satisfies your hunger. Of course, adding butter or margarine, cheese, and cream sauces to pasta and other starches will increase caloric content and transform a normally low-calorie food into one that is indeed fattening. Besides, many of these foods are high in fat and cholesterol—hardly heart-healthy! Instead, serve pasta with tomatoes or other vegetables or with clams or mussels in a light wine broth, or with a *light* sprinkling of grated parmesan cheese.

You can eat large amounts of raw or lightly processed vegetables and salads without consuming appreciable numbers of calories. Again, it's the sauces and dressings that make all the difference. Adding a rich cream or cheese sauce to a vegetable dish or salad can add hundreds of calories. Instead, use a sprinkling of lemon juice, herbs, spices, or pepper. Use only a dash of an oil-based salad dressing and avoid high-fat toppings like bacon bits or blue cheese.

Space your food intake to avoid getting too hungry. Like Sally, many overweight people will starve themselves most of the day and finally get so hungry they lose all control and end up consuming more food than they need.

Start the day with a good breakfast. Studies have found that food consumed early in the day is less likely to end up as stored body fat as food consumed at dinner or in the evening. Breakfast especially provides the energy you need to carry you through the early part of the day. Jane Brody, the *New York Times* health columnist who once had a weight problem herself, offers this advice about meal planning: "Eat like a king at breakfast, a prince at lunch, and a pauper at dinner!"

Many people think that snacks are absolute "no-nos" when it comes to weight control. Actually, many weight-control experts advise moderate snacks midway between meals to prevent excessive hunger. But the snacks should be part of your total day's meal plan and not "extras." For example, you can shift an English muffin and glass of skim milk from your breakfast menu to a midmorning snack. Similarly, you can save an item from lunch to eat during the afternoon. But be sure to include these snacks in your day's total calorie count.

Increase your physical activity. As stressed earlier, exercise is a very important aspect of long-term weight control as well as of cardiovascular conditioning. Exercise not only burns up calories, but it also prevents a slowdown in your metabolism, thus promoting long-term weight control.

Most exercise conditioning programs call for 20 to 30 minutes of vigorous aerobic exercise three or four times a week. If you are trying to lose weight, it's a good idea to exercise daily rather than on alternating days. The exercise can be moderate: a half hour's walk at a moderate pace of 3 miles an hour will burn up about 135 calories. Step up that pace to 1 mile in 15 minutes, and in a half hour, you burn up almost 200 calories. Not all physical activity is relegated to specific exercise sessions. By varying your routine only slightly, you can markedly increase your physical activity. For example, climbing just two flights of stairs a day will burn up 300 calories in a week. Walking seven city blocks at a brisk pace will use up about 60 calories. See Chapter 8 for more specific suggestions and guidelines. And always check with your doctor before embarking on an exercise program or excelerating an existing one.

Pay attention to the way you eat. Studies of overweight people have found that many have a similar way of eating. For example, they invariably eat fast, seldom pausing between bites, and are usually the first at the table to empty their plates. When you eat fast, you don't give the appetite control center in the brain a chance to "catch up" and signal a cutoff to the body's hunger signals. If you still feel hungry even though you've cleaned your plate, chances are you'll go back for seconds.

Learn to slow down. Take small bites and chew your food slowly before swallowing. Make a conscious effort to put your fork down between each bite. About midway in the meal, take a two- or three-minute breather. This will give your appetite control center more time to send out messages of satiety.

Often, we have to work at unlearning what we were taught as children. "Eat, don't talk" is a rule at many family dinner tables, yet by engaging in conversation, you will eat more slowly and run less risk of overeating. "Clean your plate" is also a common rule in many households. (Remember your mother urging you to eat every bite, and to remember all those starving children who had to go to bed with empty stomachs?) Again, forget what your mother told you—at least about those eating habits! Stop eating as soon as your hunger is satisfied, even if there is food still on your plate. Either take smaller portions to begin with or close your eyes and discard what's left.

Remove serving dishes from the table as soon as people have taken what they want. This removes the temptation to take second helpings. In any event, don't let yourself become a human garbage can by eating leftovers you can't bear to throw away or, even worse, eating what's left on the plates of others simply because you don't want to waste the food. (If you're tempted to eat rather than discard the leftovers, repeat the following to yourself until the urge passes: "A moment on the lips, and a lifetime on your hips . . .")

Start cutting calories in the shopping and preparation stages. If you find you can't resist ice cream, cookies, chips, nuts, and other high-calorie foods once they're in the house, don't buy them in the first place. Or buy them in very small quantities. Better still, look for low-calorie substitutes, and incorporate them into your overall eating plan. Table 11 (page 110) gives tips on low-calorie substitutes for your shopping cart.

Calories can be added or subtracted in the cooking process. Use a minimum of fat when cooking. Bake, roast, broil, or steam instead of sautéing or frying. Buy lean cuts of meat and then remove all visible fat. Most of the fat in poultry lies just beneath the skin. Trim away and discard all the skin and underlying fat. And don't fry the chicken in more fat!

When baking, you usually can reduce the amount of fat in a recipe by half or even more without altering the taste or texture. Depending upon the recipe, you can add a little water, skim milk, juice, or fruit to make up for the moisture in the omitted fat. Don't be afraid to experiment with your own recipes. There are a number of excellent low-fat cookbooks now on the market. (Even in these recipes, you usually can reduce the fat a bit more without losing out on taste or texture.)

Take a hard look at what you drink. Alcoholic beverages, especially those made with hard liquors, are high in calories (see Table 12, page 111). But other beverages also can contribute large numbers of calories. Many people, for example, drink fruit juices, milk, or soft drinks instead of water. If you have two glasses of orange juice, two glasses of whole milk, and two 12-ounce colas in a day—amounts that are typical for large numbers of people—you will consume about 750 to 800 calories in these drinks alone. Switching to skim milk (90 calories per cup versus 150 in whole milk) helps. Vegetable juices are lower in calories than most fruit juices. Carbonated soda or seltzer, including fruit-flavored varieties, are non caloric substitutes for regular soft drinks and excessive fruit juice. (Look for low-sodium brands if you have high blood pressure.) Water, of course, also contains no calories. Try keeping a bottle of water with slices of lemon or lime added in the refrigerator as a refreshing alternative to juice or soft drinks when you are thirsty.

Table 11. Tips on Shopping and Low-Calorie Substitutes

If you normally buy:	Substitute:
Prime cuts of beef	Choice, lean, or low-fat cuts
Frozen vegetables in butter/ cream sauces	Fresh or plain frozen
Breaded chicken, fish sticks, etc.	Plain fillets
Ritz and other cocktail crackers	Saltines, oyster crackers
Buttered popcorn	Plain and flavor it yourself
Regular mayonnaise	Low-calorie substitutes
Cheddar and other hard cheeses	Skim or part-skim cheeses
Ice cream	Ice milk, sherbert sorbet, or low-fat frozen yogurt
Pastries	Make your own (using reduced fats)
Frosted cereals	Puffed, shredded, or other low-sugar varieties
Tuna packed in oil	Water-packed brands
Whole-milk yogurt	Non-fat, plain (add your own fruit)
Regular cottage cheese	Skim or 1% fat cottage cheese
Nondairy coffee creamers	Nonfat dried milk
Fruit canned in heavy syrup	Fresh or juice-packed fruit

NOTE: This is only a small sampling of substitutes. You will find many more as you walk down the food aisles.

221111

Table 12. Approximate Caloric Content of Selected Alcoholic Beverages

Drink	Quantity	Calories
Beer (4.5% alcohol by volume)	12 oz.	151
Beer, regular	2 oz.	150
Daiquiri	1 cocktail glass	122
Eggnog, Christmas-type	4 oz.	335
Gin, rum, vodka, whiskey, 80-proof	1 ½ oz.	104
Gin, rum, vodka, whiskey, 86-proof	1 ½ oz.	112
Gin, rum, vodka, whiskey, 90-proof	1 ½ oz.	118
Manhattan	3 ½ oz.	164
Martini	3 ½ oz.	140
Tom Collins	10 oz.	180
Whiskey sour	1 cocktail	138
Wine, champagne (Dom)	4 oz.	84
Wine, dessert (18.8% alcohol)	1 wine glass	137
Wine, muscatel/port	3 ½ oz.	158
Wine, sauterne, California	3 ½ oz.	84
Wine, sherry (Dom)	2 oz.	84
Wine, table (12.2% alcohol by volume)	1 wine glass	85
Wine, vermouth, French	1 wine glass	105

Exercise prudence when eating out. Increasingly, Americans are eating more meals in restaurants, including fast-food outlets. Some studies have found that, on an average, a third or more of our meals are eaten away from home. It is possible to get low-calorie meals in restaurants, including fast-food ones, but to do so, you may need to ask questions and make requests. If your meal is being prepared to order, don't hesitate to ask that the chef not use butter or other fat to prepare it. Request that sauces and dressing be served on the side. Sometimes you can request smaller portions (often, the appetizer version is a normal at-home serving) or ask that a portion of your food be set aside to take home. (You can ask that it be divided before it is brought to the table, thus removing the temptation to overeat.)

You often can put together a wholesome and interesting main course at a salad bar—but beware of the pitfalls. Many salad bar dishes, such as pasta, rice, or meat salads, are loaded with oil or other fats. Stick with the plain raw or steamed vegetables, lean meats, and fruits, and then make your own dressing with lemon juice or vinegar and just a sprinkling of oil. Instead of blue cheese, you can add a small amount of grated parmesan or romano, which will give a cheese flavor with less fat and fewer calories.

At fast-food restaurants, avoid foods that have been breaded and fried. A plain hamburger will have fewer calories and less fat than breaded, deep-fried chicken or fish. Many fast-food restaurants now have low-calorie (or at least lower-calorie specials. Vegetarian chili is a popular example.

Don't assume that all ethnic foods are low in calories. Many are, but there also are many exceptions. In a Chinese restaurant, for example, large amounts of oil may be used in making stir-fried dishes. Steamed dishes or noodle soups are better alternatives. A broiled dish, like Indian tandoorie chicken or seafood, will be lower in calories than a curry made with cream sauce. When ordering in a restaurant, ask how a dish is prepared before ordering. A fish poached in wine, for example, will be lower in calories than one that is pan-fried in butter.

Learn to savor and enjoy your food. Eating is one of life's great pleasures, and one that should not be diminished by weight consciousness. Dr. Herbert Spiegel, a New York psychiatrist who treats many patients with weight problems, advocates eating like a gourmet. "A true gourmet plans for a meal and then savors every bite," he explains. "They will eat slowly, and use other senses, such as sight and smell, to add to their eating pleasure. I've known many gourmets, and very few of them have been overweight." Dr. Spiegel urges his patients to eat everything they desire, but to plan for it in advance. "Gourmets plan their meals, often days in advance. I've found that most people who are overweight don't eat for pleasure; they eat because they are bored or frustrated or for some other reason. In fact, they eat so fast, they don't take the time to enjoy a meal."

7 BRINGING DIABETES UNDER CONTROL

People with diabetes mellitus bear a double burden when it comes to serious health risks. Their primary disease can be life-threatening in itself. But diabetes also increases the risk of heart attacks, high blood pressure, strokes, and kidney failure. Before the discovery of insulin, the most serious form of diabetes was invariably fatal. Today, however, the outlook for people with diabetes is greatly improved; in fact, if the disease is properly controlled, it's possible to lead a full, active life free of many if not most of its complications.

One major problem encountered in minimizing the effects of diabetes revolves around the fact that, like high blood pressure, it often goes undetected until serious damage has occurred. This implies that everyone should be periodically screened for diabetes. The U.S. Prevention Services Task Force (1989) recommends screening only in pregnancy, in those with symptoms, and—maybe—for those at high risk (marked obesity, family history, and so on). More than 10 million Americans have diabetes, yet it is estimated that only half of them are aware of their disease. Margaret Sims, a forty-seven-year-old schoolteacher who was recently referred to our clinic, is a typical example. A few weeks earlier, Mrs. Sims had taken a new job and had undergone a routine insurance physical. Her electrocardiogram showed evidence of a previous silent heart attack—a finding that prompted the insurance physician to refer her to our clinic for a more extensive cardiovascular examination.

Electrocardiograms taken both while she was resting and exercising on a treadmill showed abnormalities indicating that Mrs. Sims had, indeed, suffered an earlier silent heart attack. This type of attack does not produce the usual symptoms, such as severe chest pain, but it still causes damage to the heart muscle. Routine blood tests also showed that Mrs. Sims had Type II diabetes. Other tests indicated a possible kidney problem and that her blood cholesterol was too high.

These findings came as a great surprise to Mrs. Sims, who had considered herself basically healthy despite a persistent weight problem. "I never knew you could actually have a heart attack and not know it," she said. "And I thought diabetes also had serious symptoms. Is it really possible to have such conditions and still feel fine?"

I explained that silent heart attacks are relatively common. In fact, the late A. Bartlett Giamatti, the former Yale president and commissioner of baseball whose sudden death at the age of fifty-one stunned the nation, was found to have had a previous silent heart attack. When we find evidence of a silent heart attack, the goal is to prevent a subsequent, more serious one. In Mrs. Sims's case, her risk was compounded by her diabetes. Thus, our preventive approach was to improve her cardiovascular health by controlling her diabetes.

WHAT IS DIABETES?

There are two distinct forms of diabetes mellitus. Type I, which is also called juvenile or insulin-dependent diabetes, generally begins in the first two decades of life, although it sometimes occurs in older people, too. It is the more serious form of diabetes, but fortunately is also less common, afflicting about 1 million Americans.

In Type I diabetes, the pancreas ceases to make or release insulin, the hormone essential for proper metabolism—the process of converting food into energy sources. In particular, a person with Type I diabetes is unable to utilize blood glucose (sugar), the body's major form of fuel. Most glucose comes from carbohydrates (sugars and starches). Insulin is also needed to metabolize protein and, to a lesser degree, fats. Thus, without insulin the body cannot use most of the food that is consumed.

A person with untreated Type I diabetes usually feels ravenously hungry and may consume large amounts of food, and still be starving because the body is unable to metabolize it. As glucose accumulates in the blood (hyperglycemia), it "spills over" into the urine (glycosuria). In addition to feeling hungry, the person is usually extremely thirsty and will consume huge amounts of water. In fact, the term "diabetes" is from the Greek word for fountain or syphon; "mellitus" comes from the Latin term for honey, referring to the classic symptoms—thirst and the passage of copious amounts of sweet urine—that were recognized as early as 1500 B.C. Since Type I diabetes has such distinct symptoms and progresses rather rapidly, it usually is diagnosed within a few weeks or months.

Unlike Type I diabetes, the adult form of the disease or Type II, often occurs without symptoms, at least in its early stages, and thus can go unrecognized for years. In this form of the disease, which is also called adult-onset, noninsulin-dependent, or insulin-resistant diabetes, the body still produces insulin, but is unable to use it fully. Type II diabetes usually begins after the age of forty although it, too, can occur at any age.

As with the case of Mrs. Sims, the disease often is detected during routine urine or blood tests. Or a suspicion of diabetes may be raised by the development of secondary complications, most commonly visual disturbances; decreased resistance to infections, (especially vaginal infections in women); impotence in men; poor circulation, especially in the legs; and tingling and other signs of nerve damage. And patients with diabetes have an increased incidence of hypertension, atherosclerosis, coronary artery disease, heart attacks, and sudden death. In effect, the heart, kidneys, eyes, nerves, and blood vessels all are "target" organs of diabetes.

The causes of both types of diabetes are unknown, although it appears that an inherited tendency is instrumental. The onset of Type I diabetes often follows a viral infection or some other stress, leading some researchers to believe that an autoimmune process, in which the body responds to the invading virus by destroying its own insulin-producing cells, may be involved. The onset of Type II diabetes may also follow stress or a viral infection, but more commonly, there is no obvious precipitating event that one can remember. Since more than 80 percent of people with Type II diabetes are overweight, many researchers think that obesity may play a role in its development, but excess fat alone probably is not the sole cause.

HOW DIABETES HARMS THE HEART

Since diabetes is a metabolic disease, it is not at all surprising that it affects almost every body system. Both types of diabetes have particular detrimental effects on the heart and circulatory system. Diabetic patients have a much higher cardiovascular death rate than the general population, and women are at even greater risk than men. Studies have found that the cardiovascular death rate among diabetic men is about double that of nondiabetics, but in women, it is four to six times higher than among other women. Heart disease also strikes diabetic women at an earlier age. For example, women ordinarily do not develop serious high blood cholesterol, atherosclerosis, or coronary artery disease until after menopause, but this does not hold for women with diabetes. High blood pressure also is more prevalent among diabetic women than among their male counterparts. Other major cardiovascular complications suffered by diabetic patients include:

- Increased incidence of high blood pressure.
- Increased incidence of congestive heart failure and other diseases of the heart muscle.
- Increased development of atherosclerosis.
- Increased incidence of high blood cholesterol (LDL type) and triglycerides.
- Heart attack more likely to prove fatal than for nondiabetics.
- Increased incidence of silent or undiagnosed heart attacks.
- More severe coronary artery disease; fatty deposits contain more calcium and other materials than in nondiabetics.
- More severe vascular disease of the kidneys and its filtering units, the glomerulae.

Just why people with diabetes are more susceptible to heart disease is unknown, but many researchers suspect that high levels of blood sugar are involved in some way. Thus, it follows that normalizing blood sugar may help prevent these complications. Heretofore, this has been difficult, especially with Type II diabetics, whose blood sugar levels may vary considerably without producing symptoms. New technology that allows diabetics to measure their own blood sugar makes tight control of diabetes easier than in the past.

TREATMENT OF DIABETES

Maintaining blood sugar in a normal range is the goal of treating both types of diabetes. Even in nondiabetics, levels of blood sugar vary (usually between a range of 86 and 140 milligrams per decaliter of blood) during the course of a day. Normally, blood sugar is lowest (in the range of 80 to 115 mg/dl) after a period of fasting, such as when you first get up in the morning, and it rises after eating as the ingested food is converted to glucose. Blood glucose also rises during stress as part of the body's fight-or-flight response. Exercise, during which muscles use up large amounts of glucose, lowers blood sugar levels.

Persistently elevated fasting blood sugar levels (over 140 mg/dl) establishes a diagnosis of the disease. In borderline cases, in which the fasting blood glucose is between 115 and 160 mg/dl, additional testing may be needed, especially if there are symptoms suggesting diabetes. A glucose tolerance test, in which the body's response to consuming a prescribed amount of sugar is monitored for several hours, will be done if diabetes is suspected but the fasting blood glucose levels remain in the borderline range.

Insulin injections are essential in treating Type I diabetes. Sometimes insulin will be needed by people with Type II as well, but most people with this form of the disease already produce enough insulin, and can use diet and exercise to maintain normal blood sugar levels. If these measures are insufficient, there also are medications (called oral hypoglycemic drugs) that help the body use its own insulin more efficiently.

To achieve good control over blood sugar, people with diabetes must be especially attuned to their bodies and the many factors that can cause glucose to rise or fall. People with Type I of the disease can quickly go from one extreme to the other, experiencing low blood sugar (hypoglycemia) if they take too much insulin in relation to food or exercise, or very high levels (hyperglycemia) if they don't have enough insulin to metabolize a meal.

This is where self-monitoring of blood glucose comes in. By charting responses of blood sugar levels, diabetic patients can adjust their insulin dosage to compensate for events that send glucose up or down. Some doctors emphasize self-monitoring only for their Type I diabetes patients, but others advocate it for people with Type II as well. Mrs. Sims, for example, found it particularly helpful in following her diet.

In Type II diabetes, restricting total caloric intake is what's most important. In contrast, people with Type I must carefully distribute their calories over the course of a day and also divide them precisely among carbohydrates, protein, and fats, as well as timing their insulin injections according to their meal and exercise schedule. Type II patients don't need to be as disciplined about their schedules, but they do need to cut back on their food intake. In more than 80 percent of people with Type II diabetes, this may be all that is needed to control the disease. But it's not as simple as it sounds—anyone who has attempted to lose a few pounds knows how hard reducing food intake can be, especially on a long-term basis.

Mrs. Sims freely admitted she had a weight problem; in fact, at 175 pounds she was more than 30 percent above her ideal weight of 135. When told that her diabetes could be controlled by cutting her food intake and losing weight, she was doubtful that she could adhere to this approach. "I've tried dozens of diets and none of them work for me. Wouldn't it be easier just to take insulin?" she asked.

I explained that a lack of insulin was not her problem. "Your body is making its own insulin," I explained. "Our job is make use of it, and we know that the best way to accomplish this is by cutting calories and losing weight. Increasing your exercise will also help."

As with so many patients, Mrs. Sims was very frightened to learn that not only had she suffered a previous silent heart attack, but that she also had diabetes. She recalled that her paternal grandmother had had the disease, and eventually died of kidney failure. Her father also had developed diabetes, and suffered greatly from reduced circulation in his legs before succumbing to a heart attack in his early sixties. It was clear that she had a hereditary predisposition to the disease.

Mrs. Sims had several sessions with a dietitian and diabetes educator. After two months of dieting, her blood sugar was down to normal levels and she was greatly relieved. But when she returned three months later, her weight and blood sugar both were back up to former levels. This is very common. I've seen some patients who will starve themselves for a week or so before a doctor's appointment in hopes that their blood glucose tests will be normal or near normal. But their diabetes certainly is not under control; diabetes is a disease that demands careful day-to-day management if long-term complications are to be avoided.

In Mrs. Sims's case, we decided that self-monitoring of her blood glucose at home would provide an added incentive in long-term control of her diabetes. If after a few more months of dietary treatment her blood sugar level remained too high, medication might be tried. These medications are in a family of drugs called sulfonylureas, and they are thought to work by reducing the body's resistance to insulin. Their use is controversial because of some studies that have indicated they may not decrease, and may even increase, the risk of a heart attack. For Mrs. Sims, diet was doubly important because, in addition to her high blood sugar, she also had seriously elevated cholesterol.

In the past, people with diabetes were taught to test their urine for sugar. While that is still useful in some circumstances, urine testing is not as good as actually measuring the level of glucose in the blood. For example, blood glucose can be too high without spilling over into the urine. And by the time sugar appears in the urine, blood glucose may be back to normal. The relatively recent development of devices for home monitoring of blood glucose has truly given Type I diabetes patients greater control over their lives. By home testing, a person with diabetes can determine blood sugar levels and take immediate appropriate action if they are too high or too low. In the past, this kind of testing could be done only in a doctor's office, clinic, or hospital, and even in these settings, results often were not available for several hours. Most patients with Type I diabetes now test their blood sugar daily or even more often if needed.

Self-testing lets someone with Type II diabetes see just how effective diet and exercise can be in controlling blood sugar. This may be likened to home monitoring of blood pressure by patients with hypertension. Daily testing may not be as important as in Type I diabetes, but many Type II patients find it is useful to keep a daily record of their blood sugar levels, which they can share with their doctors or diabetes educators in assessing their treatment. Figure 6 (pages 123–124) shows a sample for keeping a blood glucose diary.

Figure 6. Diary of Blood Glucose Levels

Name _____

Week of _____

Day	Time	Circumstance	Glucose Level
Monday			
Example:	7 a.m.	Before breakfast	65
Tuesday			
Wednesday			

Day	Time	Circumstance	Glucose Level
Thursday			
Friday			
Saturday			
Sunday			

For self-testing, an automated device called a glucose meter is used. Other necessary supplies are sterile needles or lancets, gauze pads or tissues, alcohol swabs, and chemically treated (reagent) strips. In the beginning, your doctor or diabetes educator will show you how to calibrate and use your particular type of glucose meter. There are a number of different types, but all use the same general principles. Most patients can master self-testing in one or two sessions. The steps to follow are:

1. Assemble your supplies (glucose meter, lancets, alcohol swabs, pads or tissue, and reagent strips).
2. Carefully wash your hands with soap and water. Don't use an alcohol swab before the test as this may alter the results.
3. Select a site from which you will draw a few drops of blood. Most people use a fingertip—the sides of the fingers are less sensitive than the pads, where nerves are concentrated.
4. Squeeze or "milk" the finger for a few seconds to stimulate blood flow. If your hands are cold, warm them first to make sure blood is near the surface.
5. Use a clean lancet to prick the site. Many people find it difficult to actually prick a finger; there are triggering devices to use that produce a quick, painless prick.
6. Wipe away the first drop of blood, especially if your hands are sweaty. Perspiration may mix with the blood and alter the results.
7. Place a small amount of blood on the reagent strip. These strips contain an enzyme and chemicals to generate different colors. The shade or color is determined by the amount of glucose in the blood sample. (Some patients compare the color on the strip with a chart to determine their approximate glucose levels. This is not as accurate as a glucose meter, and since many people with diabetes have eye problems, many doctors recommend using a meter.)
8. According to instructions for your particular type of meter, insert the reagent strip into it. The results will appear in a digital display. Make sure that the meter is properly calibrated for the type of reagent strip you are using.

EXERCISE AND DIABETES

People tend to be preoccupied with the role of diet and drugs in the management of diabetes, overlooking still another important treatment: exercise. Even before the discovery of insulin, some doctors recognized that exercise could help control blood glucose. During exercise, the muscles require extra glucose, which lowers the amount circulating in the blood. Regular exercise also may improve insulin sensitivity, which enables some people with Type I diabetes to reduce their insulin dosage, and is also beneficial for Type II.

Regular exercise has other important benefits for the diabetic patient: it improves cardiovascular function, facilitates weight control, and may help lower high blood pressure and elevated cholesterol and other lipids. But as with all other aspects of diabetes treatment, you must plan your exercise carefully to avoid excessive swings in blood glucose.

This is especially important for people with Type I of the disease. I recall the problems of a young diabetes patient. His gym class was scheduled in the late morning, just before lunch. "I'm fine for a few minutes, but then I suddenly get so weak I can hardly move," he complained. I suggested that he test his blood sugar before gym class, and see if he had enough insulin to carry him through 45 minutes of vigorous exercise. If his blood sugar was on the low side, he should drink a glass of orange juice or milk before the class, or perhaps try to switch to a class after lunch.

In general, an exercise session should be planned for times when your blood glucose is going to be high; for example, after eating. You should not exercise shortly after taking insulin. Also, exercise can alter the uptake of insulin for special areas of the body. For example, if you inject insulin in your leg and then jog, it will be absorbed into your body more quickly than if it had been injected into your arm or abdomen.

As with other aspects of diabetes treatment, regularity is important. For example, you should try to exercise at about the same time each day, rather than making it a now-and-then or weekend activity. Measuring your blood glucose before exercise and then a half hour and an hour after a session will show you exactly what effect the activity is having on your glucose levels.

THE DIABETES DIET

Misconceptions abound regarding the so-called diabetic diet. Overall, the diet recommended for people with diabetes is comparable to any prudent diet. People with Type I diabetes must be careful to distribute their calories among carbohydrates, fat, and protein, and to have frequent small meals. But it is not necessary to buy special dietetic foods or to serve separate dishes for the person with diabetes. If you doubt this, look at the sample menus developed by dietitians at the former New York Diabetes Self-Care Program (Figure 7, pages 128–129). You will note that they incorporate the very foods served regularly in homes throughout the country. For more menus, contact your local chapter of the American Diabetes Association. As with any of our volunteer health organizations, they will be happy to help you and will provide excellent literature.

Figure 7. Sample Menus Developed by Dietitians at the Diabetes Self-Care Program

BREAKFAST
Oatmeal or choice of low-sugar dry cereals
Skim milk
Whole-grain toast
Margarine
Beverage

LUNCHES
Split pea soup
Tossed salad
Whole-grain, low-fat crackers
Skim milk or beverage

OR
Sliced turkey sandwich on whole-grain bread
Tossed salad
Apple or pear
Beverage

DINNERS
Rolled flounder
Baked potato
Spinach
Cucumber salad
Orange slices
Beverage

OR
Beef and vegetable stew
Corn bread

Tossed salad
Melon
Beverage

SNACKS
Selection of:
Low-salt, low-fat crackers
Low-fat yogurt
Fresh vegetables
Popcorn, plain or flavored with chili powder
or other nonfat flavorings
Low-fat muffins
Bagels and other breads
Fresh fruits

Adapted with permission from *Living with Diabetes* by Genell J. Subak-Sharpe, Doubleday, 1985, © G. S. Sharpe Communications.

By testing blood glucose before and at intervals after a meal, it is possible to determine just what effects various foods have on blood sugar levels. Simple sugars—table sugar, sweets, and the sugar in fruit juice and milk—produce a fast and pronounced rise in blood sugar. Complex carbohydrates, especially starches and high-fiber vegetables, also raise blood glucose, but since they are metabolized more slowly than simple sugars, the rise is slower and steadier. A certain amount of protein is converted to glucose, but takes longer than complex carbohydrates to reach the bloodstream. Fats take several hours to digest and be metabolized, and only a small portion is converted to blood glucose.

It is important to work out a specific dietary regimen with a dietitian who is experienced in working with diabetic patients. Individual considerations, such as food likes and dislikes, weight, and possible concomitant problems, such as kidney disorders, high cholesterol, and obesity are important in arriving at an individual eating program. Since cardiovascular problems are common among people with both types of diabetes, many of the tenets of a heart-healthy diet are incorporated. To review, these include:

- Consume most of your calories (about 60 percent) from carbohydrates, with emphasis on starches, vegetables, and fruits. Sugars (including alcohol) should make up no more than 10 percent of your total calories.
- Fats should not comprise more than 25 or 30 percent of your total calories, and less than 10 percent should come from saturated fat.
- Limit dietary cholesterol to 300 milligrams or less per day.
- Consume only enough calories to maintain your desirable weight.

If you have special problems, such as high cholesterol or excess weight, other dietary measures will be taken into consideration and recommended. Many diabetic patients find a support group made up of people with similar problems is especially helpful. This, along with regular self-monitoring, proved to be the answer for Mrs. Sims.

"Friends had urged me to go to Weight Watchers or other programs like that," she recounted, "but somehow I never got around to it. When I learned I had diabetes, I knew I had to do something or I'd end up like my father and grandmother." The patients' support group recommended by her dietitian met twice a week at a YMCA near the school where Mrs. Sims taught. "Any doubts I had were dispelled at my first meeting," she said. "Just knowing that other people shared my concerns and problems was helpful. And everyone had specific suggestions to contribute."

Another woman who had been about the same weight as Mrs. Sims had lost 30 pounds. She had suffered a mild heart attack about four years earlier, and like Mrs. Sims, had subsequently learned that she had diabetes. She had maintained normal blood sugars for more than a year and, happily, had not suffered any further symptoms of heart disease. "She was a great inspiration and help," Mrs. Sims recounted. "She shared her menus with me, and this was a big help in getting out of my old food rut."

Mrs. Sims also had found it hard to find time to exercise every day. Her support-group friend helped solve that problem, too. Her friend's doctor had stressed exercise conditioning as part of her cardiac rehabilitation program. "She took a 30-minute walk during her lunch hour each day. I normally spent my lunch hour in the teachers' lounge or the cafeteria. Since she worked near my school, we arranged to meet at lunchtime for a daily walk."

When Mrs. Sims came back for her six-month checkup, she was enthusiastic and filled with self-confidence. "My blood sugars are absolutely normal," she assured me, and she was right. She had lost 20 pounds and wasn't worried about putting the weight back on. And perhaps most important, there was no evidence that her heart disease had progressed.

"I've changed my eating habits for good," she said. "Before, I always looked forward to treating myself by celebrating the end of a diet with a big meal of all my old favorites—cheese, pastries, hot sausages, bacon, and butter on almost everything. No wonder I regained every pound and then some! Now I know that this is the way I'm going to eat for the rest of my life. I still have everything I like, only in smaller amounts and not as often as before."

When we got the results of Mrs. Sims's other blood and urine tests, we found that her cholesterol was down by 40 mg/dl and her urine tests were normal, indicating that there had been no lasting kidney damage. This is one case I am particularly happy to describe—it illustrates a commonsense, effective way of dealing with a very common problem.

8 EXERCISE AND YOUR HEART

The millions of Americans who are caught up in today's exercise and fitness boom are by no means the first people to discover the benefits of physical activity. Back in the fifth century the Greek physician Hippocrates, the father of medicine, stated that "Speaking generally, all parts of the body which have a function, if used in moderation and exercised in labors in which each is accustomed, thereby become healthy, well developed, and age more slowly. But if unused and left idle, they become liable to disease, defective in growth, and age quickly." This is still sound medical advice. And while it may seem that everyone in this country is on an exercise kick, the fact is, there are many millions of Americans who are sedentary. Unfortunately, a large number of our children and adolescents spend many hours each day in front of a TV set, playing computer games, or engaged in other sedentary activities. The President's Council on Fitness, for example, has found that more than half of American children and adolescents are unable to pass a simple fitness test.

Many of the more than 34 million obese adults in this country can attribute at least part of their weight problem to their sedentary life-styles. Studies by Dr. Jean Mayer, the noted nutritionist and president of Tufts University, have shown that a large portion of overweight people of all ages actually eat less than their slender counterparts, but they also are more sedentary and therefore burn fewer calories.

PROVEN BENEFITS OF EXERCISE

Modern medical research has provided statistical and scientific support to back up Hippocrates's observations. Among the most extensive are the studies by Dr. Ralph S. Paffenbarger, Jr. and his colleagues at Harvard and Stanford universities, which have followed nearly 17,000 Harvard alumni, aged thirty-four to seventy-four, who attended Harvard between 1916 and 1950. In their follow-up, which extended from 1962 to 1978, the researchers found that men who burned 2,000 or more calories a week in various physical activities—walking, climbing stairs, sports, and so forth—had a 28 percent lower annual death rate (from all causes) than their more sedentary peers. The increased longevity was even more marked when the researchers looked specifically at deaths from heart attacks and other cardiovascular diseases. In this category, the men who exercised at the 2,000-calorie-a-week level had a 39 percent lower death rate. These benefits were independent of other risk factors, such as smoking and high blood pressure. In all, the highest death rates were among smokers and sedentary men.

Other studies have pinpointed specific benefits of exercise. Researchers at the Duke University Preventive Approach to Cardiology (DUPAC) program have found that exercise

conditioning hastens recovery from a heart attack and provides important psychological benefits. When combined
with weight control and reduced salt intake, exercise may
also help lower high blood pressure, and as noted in the last
chapter, it also improves control of diabetes.

People who exercise regularly often find they have a re-
newed sense of vigor and well-being, and can cope better
with stress. Many patients even say that exercise gives them a
new, positive outlook on life. One patient summed up her
benefits of exercise this way: "I just have a much better
feeling about myself. And it is reinforced every time I look in
the mirror. I like looking at this trim new me instead of the
sagging, flabby me of a few months ago!"

In addition to documenting that exercise may help prevent
premature death, the Harvard alumni study showed that
even a moderate amount of exercise will increase longevity.
Heretofore, many exercise enthusiasts have stressed "going
for the burn" or "the no pain, no gain" approach. This study
shows that it's not necessary to jog 20 miles a week or engage
in a tremendous amount of strenuous exercise. For example,
increasing total walking from 3 to 9 miles or more a week (or
its equivalent in other activities) was sufficient to lower the
death rate by more than 25 percent.

That comes as very welcome news to many of my
patients, especially those who are middle-aged and find that
their knees can't take jogging, aerobic dancing, or other such
activities favored by younger exercisers. Jeff Allen, the fifty-
one-year-old hospital administrator you met in Chapter 2, is
a case in point. Jeff was referred to our clinic because of his
high blood pressure. He conceded that he rarely exercised
except for a weekend game of golf at his club. Even then, he
rode around the course on a cart rather than walk. I suggested
that he increase his exercise as part of a total health-
improvement plan. He agreed that this was a sound

approach, and like many businessmen, he immediately joined a health club that caters to executives.

During one of his follow-up visits, I asked Jeff how his exercise program was going. He looked a bit sheepish. "For the first few weeks, I went to the club faithfully three times a week," he said. "Then I pulled a muscle in my back and was laid up for a couple of weeks. I've been back a couple of times, but it's so hard to find the time . . ."

This is an all too familiar refrain. Many people start out with enthusiasm and the best of intentions, but after a few weeks, most backslide into their former sedentary way of life. Often the problem is picking the wrong type of exercise. I've had dozens of patients take up jogging, then later admit that they find it boring and even painful. Others will buy all sorts of expensive exercise equipment, which soon is relegated to a corner in the basement or is turned into a clothes rack. Many like Jeff will join an exercise club and then find out that it's either inconvenient or not to their taste—they may not like the routines, the loud music, the surroundings, or exercising in the presence of others.

Still others will pick an activity that requires special skills or facilities. Tennis, horseback riding, swimming, and cross-country skiing are examples of activities that provide good exercise, but may be difficult to sustain if you lack the know-how or easy access to them. So before you embark on an exercise program, find an activity that you enjoy and that is within your budget and physical capabilities.

BASICS OF EXERCISE CONDITIONING

Let's assume that, like Jeff Allen, Margaret Sims, and other patients in this book, you have decided it's time to get in shape by increasing your exercise. As is often said, while there's no absolute guarantee that physical activity will add years to your life, it's safe to say it can add life to your years. Even people who are otherwise healthy find that being in poor physical condition is limiting. Jeff Allen confided that he felt winded after climbing a flight of stairs or running a block to catch his bus. Margaret Sims had difficulty keeping up with her pupils on a school outing, and often felt physically "wiped out" by five p.m. Both spent most of their evenings sitting in front of the television, too tired to do anything more taxing or interesting.

In contrast, people who are physically fit simply have more energy and endurance. Physical fitness is defined as having enough endurance to exercise at or near your cardiovascular or biological potential. Technically, this is expressed as multiples of resting metabolism, or METS. Even at rest, your body requires a certain amount of energy to carry on its vital functions like breathing and circulation—this is called resting metabolism. Your level of physical fitness is determined by the number of METS you can comfortably sustain during exercise. Generally speaking, physically fit adults can sustain 10 to 15 METS, or exercise at 10 to 15 times their minimum energy expenditure while resting. A well-conditioned athlete usually can exercise at 20 METS, but someone who is basically sedentary and in poor physical condition may be able to sustain only 4 or 5. In practical terms, this means that you would feel out of breath after climbing one or two flights of stairs, swimming one or two laps, or walking three or four blocks at a brisk pace. For such a person, the goal of exercise conditioning would be to improve endurance to the point where you could, for example, walk a mile in 20 minutes or cycle the distance in 5 minutes without feeling tired.

It doesn't take long to begin to notice improved stamina following exercise conditioning: endurance improves measurably after even a week or two of regular exercise training. You will be able to walk farther and at a brisker pace without having your heart rate speed up so much or feeling so out of breath. This rapid improvement in stamina is due to an increased efficiency in your body's ability to use available oxygen. Two important changes occur during exercise conditioning: (1) your blood increases its capacity to carry oxygen; and (2) physically fit muscles can extract more oxygen from the blood. When you are resting, only about 30 percent of the oxygen that circulates through the body via the bloodstream is actually extracted and used. During exercise, however, more than 75 percent of the available oxygen can be extracted—this is referred to as the maximal oxygen uptake, and it is what really determines your endurance limits.

Your heart also becomes more efficient during exercise conditioning. The heart is made up mostly of muscle, and all muscles grow stronger with exercise. Specifically, as the heart's muscle strength improves, it can pump out more blood with each beat. That is why athletes and other people who are physically fit commonly have a slower heart rate than their more sedentary peers. To get an idea of what this means in terms of how hard your heart works, consider that if your heart rate were to be reduced by just five beats per minute, in a year, it would save 2.5 million beats.

This reduced heart rate does not necessarily mean that the heart will last longer, but it does mean that the heart muscle itself will be better nourished. For example, each beat or contraction of the heart muscle momentarily interrupts blood flowing through the coronary arteries. A slower heart rate means that there is more time during which the heart muscle can extract oxygen and other nutrients from its own blood supply. Thus, even if the coronary arteries are narrowed due to atherosclerosis, exercise conditioning can help improve blood flow to the heart muscle. In addition, exercise conditioning promotes the development of collateral circulation—extra blood vessels to nourish heart muscle. Thus, if a major coronary artery is seriously narrowed, collateral blood vessels can ease the burden by carrying blood that normally would flow through the larger vessels.

In order to achieve this conditioning effect, the exercise should be of sufficient intensity to push the heart rate into a target training range. Exercise physiologists and cardiologists at Duke University Medical Center have developed a prototype exercise conditioning program for heart patients. They advocate a training range of 65 to 75 percent of your maximum attainable heart rate. For practical purposes, you can estimate your safe maximum heart rate by subtracting your age from 220. The result should be within 12 beats of your maximum. Thus, if you are 40 years old, your maximum heart rate would be 180 plus or minus 12, or 168 to 192.

For a healthy person, the heart training range can be estimated by using the formula 65 to 75 percent of 220 beats per minute minus your age. For example, if you are 40 years old, you would calculate your training range as follows:

$$220 - 40 = 180 \times 65\% = 117$$
$$220 - 40 = 180 \times 75\% = 135$$

**Your training range would then
be 117 to 135 beats per minute.**

Some exercise physiologists urge a higher training rate, for example, 70 to 85 percent of your safe maximum range. This may be appropriate for people with no cardiovascular risk factors, but since this book is directed largely to people who have some risk factors, I advocate a somewhat lower range.

To achieve cardiovascular conditioning, then, your exercise should be vigorous enough to increase your heartbeat into your target training range. To have a training effect, this heart rate should be sustained for 20 to 30 minutes at a time, three or more times a week—preferably with nonexercise days between.

In the beginning, you may want to shorten the exercise sessions to 5 or 10 minutes, and gradually work up to the 20 to 30 minutes as you become more conditioned. It doesn't take long, however, to notice an improvement. Most people will find that their endurance improves after a week or so of regular exercise.

SHOULD YOU HAVE A CHECKUP FIRST?

Almost everyone can undertake some sort of exercise conditioning. I've seen heart-attack patients who could barely walk across the room before conditioning gain a new lease on life in exercise rehabilitation programs. I recall one person who was so out of shape he was panting after climbing a flight of stairs, work up to running a marathon. I'm not advocating that you set your sights on a marathon, but unless you are severely disabled, you certainly should be able to enjoy a half hour or so of brisk walking without feeling tired.

Before undertaking exercise training, however, you should check with your doctor, who may recommend that you have an exercise tolerance test first. This test involves exercising on a treadmill, stationary bicycle, or set of stairs while you are hooked up to an electrocardiograph (ECG) machine. Your heart's function will be monitored as you increase the intensity of exercise. The test may be stopped at any time, but unless problems occur, it usually is continued until your heart rate reaches a predetermined level or until you are too tired to continue. For people with heart disease or cardiovascular risk factors, an exercise tolerance test is particularly useful in determining safe parameters for an exercise conditioning program.

Not everyone needs an exercise tolerance test before beginning a physical conditioning program, however. If you are under the age of thirty-five, are basically healthy, and have no cardiovascular risk factors, then you probably can begin an exercise program without a tolerance test. Put another way, an exercise tolerance test is recommended for anyone over thirty-five who heretofore has been sedentary. It also is recommended before exercise conditioning, regardless of age, if you fall into a high-risk group for a heart attack. Specific indications for a preconditioning exercise tolerance test include:

■ A previous heart attack or diagnosis of coronary artery disease.

■ High blood pressure.

■ A history of cardiovascular symptoms, such as irregular heartbeats or chest pains (angina pectoris).

■ High blood cholesterol.

■ Cigarette smoking.

■ Diabetes mellitus.

■ Obesity.

■ A strong family history of heart disease or premature death (for example, a parent who had a heart attack before the age of fifty).

Using the results of your exercise tolerance test, your doctor can then give you a specific exercise prescription, spelling out your target heart rate and outline how often and how long you should exercise.

START WITH WALKING

Of course, most people do not need a formal exercise prescription to undertake a conditioning program. All you really need are common sense and a determination to improve your physical fitness. Once you start to exercise regularly, chances are you will enjoy your new found sense of vigor and wellbeing so much that you won't need any urging to keep it up. Patients often ask me what kind of exercise is best. For my money, you can't beat walking for good, all-round exercise. Walking exercises almost all your large muscles, especially if you add the pumping arm motion of fitness walking. It requires no special equipment except comfortable, properly fitting shoes. You don't need a special place; a park, city sidewalks, along a country road, even a shopping-mall parking lot all are suitable places for walking. You can walk by yourself or with friends or family members. You can fit walking into even the most hectic schedule. For example, you can walk part of the way to or from work.

To achieve a conditioning effect, you should walk at a pace brisk enough to increase your heart rate into your training zone. In general, this entails walking at a pace of 3 to 4 miles an hour. To make sure you are in your training zone, take your pulse before exercising and then stop momentarily to take it again after you reach your full stride. By now, your heart rate should have increased to your target level, and you can continue walking (or doing other exercise) at that level. After a few sessions, you should be able to tell just by the way you feel whether your heart rate has increased sufficiently.

SPECIAL CAUTIONS

Moderation is the key to success in exercise conditioning. Almost all exercise-related injuries can be prevented by using common sense. The "no pain, no gain" approach to exercise is increasingly being discredited. Exercise should be pleasurable, not painful. Make "train instead of strain" your motto. There is no added benefit in exercise conditioning beyond your target zone; nor is there any added conditioning benefit in exercising more than 30 minutes in a session. The longer you exercise, the more calories you burn up, which may be a plus if you are trying to lose weight. But you also increase your risk of joint and muscle problems.

If you experience pain of any kind while exercising, stop! Trying to jog through a leg pain increases the likelihood of joint or muscle injuries. Other types of pain may be a warning sign of a heart problem or other serious disorder. If you experience any of the following while exercising, you should stop and consult your doctor:

■ Chest pain or pain spreading to the jaws, arm, back, or mouth.
■ Excessive fatigue or shortness of breath.
■ Dizziness or feeling faint.
■ Irregular heartbeat or a feeling of "flipflop" in your chest.
■ Unusual or severe pain in a joint or muscle.
■ Recurring or continuing muscle cramps.
■ Nausea or vomiting.
■ Headache.
■ Prolonged (more than 10 minutes) increase in your heart rate after stopping exercising.
■ Unusual back pain.
■ Development of leg cramps (particularly, if not experienced before).

Use common sense in regard to the weather when you exercise. For example, when it is hot and muggy, plan your walk or other exercise session for the early morning or evening, rather than during the hottest time of the day. Dress appropriately. Expose as much skin as possible when it's hot and humid, and no matter what the weather, don't exercise in a rubber suit that holds in body heat and perspiration. Drink plenty of water before and after you exercise, especially if it is hot and humid and you perspire a good deal. Avoid taking salt pills: extra water should be all you need to restore lost fluids.

9 IS STRESS REALLY A RISK FACTOR?

We often hear people say, "He's working himself to death!" or, "He gets so angry, I'm afraid he'll have a heart attack." In fact, whenever a person falls ill, especially with a heart attack or stroke, people often seek an explanation in the areas of personality and stress rather than other, more established risk factors. The ancient physicians associated "apoplexy"—the early term for a stroke, which also could have been sudden death from a heart attack—with anger and stress. Sir William Osler, the famed Johns Hopkins physician who is often called the father of modern medicine, believed there was a link between stress and heart disease. In 1897, he wrote: "In the worry and strain of modern life, arterial degeneration is not only very common, but develops often at a relatively early age. For this I believe that the high pressure at which men live and the habit of working the [human] machine to its maximum capacity, are responsible rather than excess in eating and drinking."

Today, people widely believe that there is a strong relationship between emotions and health. I've had many patients who are convinced that stress brought on their heart attacks. Retrospective (after the fact) studies have found that many heart attack victims recently encountered particularly stressful life events—job loss, retirement, death of a loved one. And this relationship has also been associated with aggravation of angira, control of high blood pressure, and even the development of malignant hypertension.

Still, there are many doubters in the medical community. Until recently, we had little hard evidence regarding stress and health. For one thing, the physical associations with stress per se are not as easy to measure as, for example, those of high blood pressure, cholesterol, or cigarette smoking. Also, there is no single definition of stress—what one person considers unbearable stress may be pure pleasure to another.

ARE YOU A "TYPE A"?

Through a number of scientific studies, we are beginning to understand better the possible role of stress or, more accurately, our response to stress, in heart disease. Some twenty years ago, two San Francisco researchers, Drs. Meyer Friedman and Raymond Rosenman, correlated Type A personality with an increased risk of heart attacks. According to their studies, Type A personality characteristics include aggressiveness, hostility, excessive anger, and preoccupation with time and success—many of the traits common among people our society considers "successful." Friedman and Rosenman proposed that the Type A personality be added to the list of cardiovascular risk factors. In general, such people's response to stress is more pronounced and negative than that of the less driven and calmer Type B's.

A number of other researchers began to study the possible link between personality and heart disease. Dr. Redford B. Williams Jr. and his colleagues at Duke University Medical Center administered personality tests to more than 2,000 patients undergoing coronary angiography—special X-ray studies of the heart's blood vessels. They found that younger Type A patients had more severe coronary artery disease than their Type B counterparts, but the correlation did not seem to hold among older men. In these older patients, people with Type B personality traits had some severe disease. The Duke researchers attributed this to survival factors. "We concluded," Dr. Williams recently explained, "that by the age of fifty-five or so, the Type A's were no longer around. They already had succumbed to a heart attack."

The Duke researchers also obtained hormonal studies, and found that men with Type A personality tended to have higher levels of catecholamines, which include adrenaline (noradrenaline) and other so-called stress hormones which are released as part of the body's fight or flight response. These findings led those investigators to hypothesize that people with Type A personality were "hyperresponders" to stress, and that their overreaction might in some way be involved in initiating high blood pressure, elevated cholesterol, and other heart-attack risk factors. But even so, Type A personality was not as strong a predictor of heart disease as the traditional risk factors, such as cigarette smoking or cholesterol.

Still, as Dr. Williams recounts, "There's something about Type A behavior that is associated with more severe coronary disease in our younger patients." Of course, heart attacks are by no means limited to people with Type A personality, and many Type A's are free of heart disease. And not all Type A's are alike; certain characteristics that predominate in some are absent in others. Thus, Dr. Williams and other researchers began to look at specific aspects of Type A behavior to see if some characteristics are more detrimental than others. When ranking individual risk factors, Williams and his colleagues found that people with high levels of hostility, anger, cynicism, and mistrust had a higher incidence of heart attacks than Type A people who were not so likely to respond to stress with anger and hostility. These people may be just as competitive and time-driven as their heart attack–prone peers, but they are more trusting and less hostile and angry. In fact, they found that their younger (aged 25 to 50) Type A patients who were characterized as being angry, hostile, and mistrusting had a fivefold increased risk of dying.

What advice does Dr. Williams have for these Type A's? Strive to control your anger and hostility by becoming more trusting and less cynical. Even if further research disproves any link between heart disease and anger, hostility, mistrust and cynicism, there's no doubt that overcoming these negative personality traits can make life much more enjoyable. The following are tips for overcoming your anger and hostility:

Voice your anger and then forget it. Everyone gets angry now and then. Rather than seething in silence, it's better to express your feelings in as calm and rational a manner as possible, and then put the incident behind you. Don't let your anger fester until you "blow up."

Find alternative outlets for your hostility. Instead of taking out your ill feelings on colleagues or family members, find an activity that will allow you to express your hostility without harming others and yourself. For example, some people work out their hostilities by exercising. Others have been helped by joining support groups. Going on periodic wilderness retreats, such as those of Outward Bound, or engaging in similar activities that force you to focus on surviving on your own in a strange environment, can help gain new perspectives.

Take time now and then to have fun. It's surprising how many otherwise successful people admit that they seldom if ever do anything "just for the fun of it." We all need time and activities that permit decompression.

Investigate new stress-coping techniques. Possibilities include yoga, meditation, daily relaxation exercises, and biofeedback training. How about reading something unrelated to your work? Schedule time away from your phone, mail, and job. Any of these can be used to divert feelings of anger or hostility.

Avoid situations that invariably make you angry. If, for example, standing in line at the bank always irritates you, try banking by machine or mail, or going to the bank at a less crowded time.

Make a conscious effort to be more trusting. If you feel that "everyone's out to get me," something is wrong. Psychological counseling may be helpful. Simply confiding in a friend or family member also can help overcome feelings of distrust.

Try to focus on admirable qualities in others. It's easy to stay angry if you constantly dwell on others' shortcomings and faults. Very few people are all bad—or all good, for that matter. Look for and foster the positive instead of concentrating on people's faults.

THE LONELY HEART

Another stress-related area involves the possible effects of loneliness or social isolation on heart disease. As with Type A personality, the evidence to date is inconclusive, but it is

convincing enough to prompt some researchers to suggest
social isolation as a possible factor in heart disease and other
illnesses.

In many respects, social support is even harder than personality traits to define. In attempting to define social isolation, social scientists point to a range of concepts that include
social networks (friends, family members, and others with
whom you can talk and share experiences and problems) and
a feeling of belonging (for example, a family structure,
church or club memberships, and the like). A number of
epidemiological studies have found that people with high
levels of social support have a lower rate of heart attacks than
those lacking in this area. The differences persist even after
taking other cardiovascular risk factors into account. For
example, a study of more than 3,800 Japanese-American men
in San Francisco found that those who lacked in social affilia-
tion (no family members or strong social ties) had an increased incidence of heart attacks, independent of age,
physical activity, or family history of heart disease.

Several studies suggest that social support and networks
may be more important for men than for women. For example, a large-scale study of mortality from all causes in
Tecumseh, Michigan, found that being single and/or lacking
involvement in organizations and leisure activities correlated
with a higher death rate in men. Interestingly, this did not
necessarily hold for women: the researchers found a statistical
correlation only between church attendance and mortality
among women. Similarly, a study involving 13,300 men and
women in North Karelia, Finland, found that men in the
lowest quarter of the social network index had twice the
overall mortality and 1.8 times the death rate from heart
attacks compared to men in the highest quarter. Again, these
findings did not hold up for women.

A high level of social support also has been linked to an increased likelihood of surviving a heart attack. A follow-up study of some 2,500 male heart attack victims found that those who were socially isolated and were in stressful circumstances, or who had difficulty coping with stress, were four times more likely to die than those with lower stress levels and better social networks.

In a related area, several studies have correlated a lack of job control with an increased risk of heart attacks. People who hold jobs that make high demands over which the worker has little control have a higher death rate than people who have more control over their situation. Studies have found, for example, that postal workers who have a demanding job, but very little or no control over their work load, procedures, or environment, have a higher than average incidence of heart attacks. A large-scale Swedish study, involving 13,779 men and women, found a relationship between heart disease and jobs with high demand, low control, and low social support. Perhaps it is the frustration in the lack of ability to control the situation around you that promotes stress. Think of the tieup in traffic, the airline delays, the snags at work or at home that add to your level of stress.

Exactly how these various factors affect the heart is unknown, but they seem to be independent of other risk factors. It's interesting to note that men seem to be more vulnerable than women. This may be attributed to the fact that women often are better at "networking" and developing social contacts than men. From an early age in our society, girls are encouraged to look to (and after) others, to join in group play, and to express their feelings and desires. In contrast, men are expected to be independent and strong— the rugged John Wayne type of individualism. Fortunately, these stereotypes are falling as new roles and expectations evolve for both genders.

While things like social isolation and on-the-job stresses may sometimes seem to be beyond our control, in reality, there's a good deal we could do to overcome them. It's often noted that the world is full of lonely people; the task is to bring them together. A good starting point is to find an interest outside your job and then link up with others who have similar interests. The possibilities are limitless. Check the listing of adult education classes at your local high school or college. YMCAs, churches, community action groups, employee organizations, business or professional groups, and craft or hobby clubs or classes are among the dozens of possible sources for networking. I recall one patient whose job took him to a new city where he was a total stranger. "I spent a few months feeling bored and sorry for myself," he said, "and then decided that it was up to me to get out and find some new friends." He looked over the list of adult classes being offered by a nearby community college, and decided to sign up for one in bread baking. "My idea of cooking was to pop a frozen dinner in the microwave, but something about making bread interested me."

The class was small—only about seven or eight others, with men predominating. One of his fellow would-be bakers had gone to the same college, and although they were in different classes, they remembered many of the same professors and facets of college life. They had dinner together a couple of times, and through his new acquaintance, he began to meet other people. Before long, he started to feel more at home, and that he "belonged." "It's making that first move that's hard," he recalled recently.

Another patient, a salesman who traveled a good deal, always sought out square-dancing groups in new cities. "I know I can always count on meeting people with a shared interest," he said, "and an evening of relaxing yet vigorous fun."

If it's true that an isolated, lonely heart is more vulnerable to disease, making that first move may be life-saving. In any event, it's better than feeling cut off and isolated.

10 PUTTING TODAY'S MEDICINE TO WORK FOR YOU

Almost daily, there's more good news for people who are at high risk for a heart attack. Over the last two decades, the death rate from heart attacks and other forms of heart disease has fallen by more than a third. The decline in strokes has been even more pronounced—down by more than a half.

Unquestionably, our changing life-style can be credited for a large part of this decrease. There is mounting evidence that putting into practice the steps to lower cardiovascular risk factors described in this book pays off in terms of longer, healthier lives. But advances in medicine have also played a major role in cutting the death rate. Thus, it's important that you know about these advances and when you should use them—indeed, using a combination of risk-factor reduction and medical advances constitutes the best approach to improving your odds of avoiding or surviving a heart attack. Although a detailed discussion of these numerous medical advances is beyond the scope of this book, this chapter will describe some of the newest and most important.

NEW DIAGNOSTIC PROCEDURES

Just a few decades ago, physicians had to rely mostly on their experience, a stethoscope, blood pressure and electrocardiographic machines, and conventional X rays to diagnose heart disease. While these still remain crucial diagnostic tools, today's physician also can turn to a variety of space-age "high-tech" or "biotech" advances to obtain a much more accurate and complete picture of the art. These techniques include:

Cardiac catheterization and angiography. These procedures allow your doctor to visualize the heart, its blood vessels, and other structures. The catheter—a thin, flexible tube—is inserted into either the venous or arterial systems through a small incision in the arm or the groin, and then passed to the heart or desired blood vessel. Once the catheter is in place, an inert dye (contrast material) is injected directly into the heart, coronary arteries, or other vessel. This dye makes the heart's structures and blood vessels visible on X rays, and by using this test, a physician can pinpoint exactly any areas of blockage or other abnormalities. For example, catheterization and angiography are done to locate areas of narrowed coronary arteries before bypass surgery or angioplastic therapy (see below).

Angioplasty. This procedure converts the diagnostic technique of catheterization into treatment. It is accomplished by inserting a balloon-tipped catheter into the artery and advancing it to the area where the vessel is clogged by fatty deposits. The balloon is then inflated, which flattens fatty deposits occluding the artery and widens the vessel opening, allowing normal blood flow.

Sometimes angioplasty is done while a heart attack is in process. Clot-dissolving drugs (thrombolytic agents) are then injected via the catheter directly into the coronary clot (thrombus), and the balloon is then inflated to widen the artery opening.

Echocardiography. This test uses sound waves to create a map of the heart. It has several distinct advantages: it is safe, painless, and noninvasive, and it allows a doctor to observe the heart while it is in motion. During echocardiography, a device called a transducer, which gives off high-frequency sound waves and receives back their echo signals, is passed over the chest. The echoes are fed into a computer, which translates them into an image that is projected onto a screen and recorded simultaneously on a chart. Echocardiography is particularly useful in assessing heart size, chamber wall thicknesses, and the shape of any abnormalities of the heart valves. Since it is noninvasive and does not use radiation, it permits assessment of heart structure and function.

Doppler ultrasonography is a variation in which sound waves are used to study blood flow through the heart and major blood vessels.

Heart scans (scintigraphy). These tests entail injecting a small amount of diagnostic (not therapeutic) radioactive material (radioisotope) into the bloodstream and following its progress through the heart and its structures. There are three different kinds of heart scans. A technetium scan is done within hours of a suspected heart attack and is used to detect areas of heart-muscle death. With a thallium scan, the isotope is injected during an exercise tolerance (treadmill or bicycle) test. It is used to determine whether areas of heart muscle are receiving enough blood supply, and hence adequate oxygen, during physical activity. In a gated-blood pool scan, red blood cells are labeled with technetium, a radioactive substance, and then injected into a vein and followed to observe how well the heart is pumping blood through each of its chambers and out into the aorta. This latter technique permits another means for assessing the function of the heart.

Magnetic resonance imaging (MRI). This test uses a strong magnetic field to make the atoms of the body generate energy waves that create a three-dimensional image of body tissues. It is relatively new and is particularly useful in examining the brain after a suspected stroke or injury. Although it is not as useful as some other tests for examining organs such as the heart which are constantly in motion, it may be used to detect cardiac inflammation and other abnormalities.

Positron emission tomography (PET) scans. This technique, which is still in its infancy, uses special radioactive chemicals which are injected through a vein, and then monitored with special tracers to study the metabolism of the heart's muscle. Since the technique requires extremely costly equipment, its use is now limited to institutions carrying out research on diseases of the heart muscle.

Heart enzyme tests. These are blood studies that measure levels of various circulating muscle enzymes. After a heart attack, the injured cardiac muscle "leaks out" certain enzymes from the damaged cells. Thus an elevation in cardiac muscle enzymes can be useful for diagnosing a heart attack and to predict the extent of heart muscle damage. The greater the amount of circulating enzymes, the more extensive and severe is the injury or heart attack.

24-hour ECG and blood pressure tests. These tests are designed to provide information about the heart's rhythm or blood pressure over a period of time. A 24-hour electrocardiogram (ECG) entails carrying a cassette size electrocardiograph machine, also called a Holter monitor, that is attached to leads positioned in various places on the chest. The purpose is to produce a continuous recording of the heart's electrical activity. This record, in the form of an ECG strip, is later analyzed by computer for abnormal heart rhythms and other abnormalities that may not show up during a conventional ECG in a doctor's office.

The 24-hour blood pressure measurement works on the same principle. A blood pressure cuff is placed on the arm, and blood pressure is measured and recorded every few minutes over a time period. Sometimes the ECG and blood pressure recordings are done simultaneously.

A host of new medications provide some of our most dramatic advances against heart disease. In addition, both heart attacks and strokes are being prevented by putting old drugs, including ordinary aspirin, to new uses. The following are some of the medications that are revolutionizing the treatment of heart disease.

ANTICLOTTING DRUGS

Normally, blood clots form only in response to a cut or some other injury. For reasons that still are not fully understood, people with atherosclerosis are especially vulnerable to the formation of clots at the site of the fatty deposits. A heart attack occurs when a clot blocks a coronary artery (a coronary thrombosis); a stroke occurs when a clot blocks a blood vessel in the brain (cerebrovascular thrombosis). Drugs that are used to prevent blood clotting have been termed "blood-thinning" agents.

Fibrinolytic agents. New drugs that can actually dissolve these clots are capable of reversing the clot obstruction that is producing a heart attack or stroke, and thereby preventing much of the damage to vital organs. Two of the most widely used are streptokinase and the newer tissue-type plasminogen activator (TPA). When given within the first few hours of a heart attack, they can restore normal coronary blood flow and prevent the death of heart muscle. The drugs are sometimes administered at the same time as balloon angioplasty, which seems to reduce the risk of new clot formation.

Antiplatelet drugs. These are drugs that inhibit or retard clot formation. Platelets are circulating blood cells that clump together to promote the formation of blood clots. Antiplatelet drugs lower the "stickiness" of platelets, thereby preventing them from clumping and propagating other cells to form clots that obstract the flow of blood. Aspirin is the most common example of an antiplatelet drug. Recent studies have found that men who take a very small amount of aspirin (a half tablet or one baby aspirin every other day is sufficient) can reduce their risk of a heart attack. It is possible that low-dose aspirin may also lower the risk of thrombotic stroke. Caution should be used in taking aspirin, however. Excessive blood thinning may promote serious internal bleeding. It also may cause a hemorrhagic stroke, especially in a person who has high blood pressure and weakened blood vessels.

Other, more powerful anticlotting (anticoagulant) drugs include heparin, warfarin, and dicumarol. These are potent drugs that often are used in a hospital setting or for special problems that increase clot formation. For example, one of these anticlotting drugs may be given after heart valve surgery to prevent clotting. Careful monitoring is required to prevent excessive blood thinning, which can result in hemorrhaging.

DRUGS TO IMPROVE HEART FUNCTION

Many drugs that improve heart function have multiple benefits. For example, several drugs are capable of easing angina, lowering blood pressure and preventing rhythm disturbances. Classes of heart drugs include:

Antiarrhythmic medications. There are many types of abnormal heart rhythms (arrhythmia or dysrhythmia), and, fortunately, most are minor and do not require treatment. Some, however, may lead to serious, even life-threatening disruptions in the heart's normal beating. Digitalis, which makes the heart beat more slowly and forcefully, is one of the oldest drugs in this class, but it has been assisted by the addition of newer drugs that control heart rhythm. These include beta blockers and calcium channel blockers, which have the added beneficial effects of lowering blood pressure and treating angina, and others that are more powerful and more specific in the ability to restore normal heart rhythm. Since sudden death may often result from rhythm disturbances rather than diseased blood vessels, diagnosing and treating cardiac arrhythmias may be life-saving.

Anti-anginal medications. Angina pectoris is the medical name for chest pains that occur when the heart muscle is not getting enough oxygen or its demand is increased so much that the blood supply cannot keep pace. Angina usually is caused by narrowed coronary arteries, but in some cases it may be due to a coronary artery spasm, a condition called variant angina. Nitroglycerin has long been used to ease angina by dilating the coronary arteries. Newer antianginal drugs, such as beta blockers and calcium antagonists, are prescribed both to treat and prevent attacks of angina. Some studies indicate that these medications also may help prevent certain recurrent heart attacks.

Antihypertensive medications. There are now a wide array of drugs used to lower blood pressure. As stressed in Chapter 4, these medications enable us to control blood pressure with a minimum of adverse side effects. Specific classes of antihypertensive drugs include diuretics, direct-acting vasodilators, beta blockers, calcium channel antagonists, and ACE (angiotensin converting enzyme) inhibitors, centrally acting drugs, and drugs that inhibit the sympathetic nervous system.

Cholesterol-lowering medications. For many people with high levels of blood cholesterol, diet and weight reduction are all that is needed. Others, however, require medication, and there now are a number of effective cholesterol-lowering drugs with different mechanisms of action. Some, such as cholestyramine and colestipol, are not absorbed from the digestive tract. Instead, they bind with bile salts, which contains large amounts of cholesterol, and are excreted in the stool. This prevents the bile salts and cholesterol from being returned to the liver and bloodstream.

Other cholesterol-lowering drugs work through the liver, where most of the body's cholesterol is manufactured. Niacin (nicotinic acid) in high doses is one of the oldest and most effective drugs in this category. Gemfibrosil reduces cholesterol levels, but is more effective in lowering triglyceride levels; it also may elevate HDL cholesterol levels. The recently released lovastatin works by reducing the synthesis of cholesterol (see Chapter 5).

Many of these cardiovascular drugs are truly life-saving; others have enabled people whose activities had been severely limited by heart disease to resume active, productive lives. It should be stressed, however, that any drug that affects your heart's function must be taken with great care. Follow your doctor's instructions and be sure to return for regular checkups. If you encounter problems that you think are related to a medication, check with your doctor as soon as possible. Above all, do not alter your dosage, or start or stop a medication, without first checking with your doctor. For example, some drugs, such as beta blockers, require gradual tapering off rather than stopping abruptly.

NEW SURGICAL PROCEDURES AND TREATMENTS

Surgery continues to play an increasingly important role in treating heart disease. When I started my medical career, operating on the heart was done—but rarely. One of the earliest heart operations, developed by pioneering doctors at Johns Hopkins, was designed to improve the blood flow of "blue babies," youngsters born with multiple congenital heart defects. At the time, this operation was considered a modern miracle, because it involved operating on the heart while it was beating. Then came the development of the heart-lung machine, which maintains a patient's vital circulation to the brain and other organs while the heart is stopped. This allows a surgeon to operate on a still heart without worrying about keeping blood flowing to other organs. And it would never have been possible without modern techniques of blood typing and blood banking.

Today, operations including heart valve and blood vessel replacement, repair of serious congenital defects, and coronary and other vessel bypasses, are commonplace. In some institutions, even heart transplants are almost routine. The concept and surgical knowhow for the heart transplant has been with us for several decades, but it was not until the development of new drugs that suppress the body's immune system and its rejection of the transplanted organs, that the operations became routine.

Some types of abnormal cardiac rhythms now can be cured surgically. For example, some dysrhythmias are caused by electrical impulses generated from foci of abnormal heart muscle. Heretofore, these abnormal rhythms required life-long drug therapy. Today, many people can be cured by first mapping the electrical activity of the heart to locate the abnormal area, then surgically cutting through it to prevent transmission of the abnormal electrical impulses.

Rapidly advancing medical research promises even more dramatic treatments for heart disease. One experimental area involves combining angioplasty and lasers—concentrated beams of light—to dissolve, rather than simply flatten, the fatty deposits as in the present balloon angioplasty. To date, most of the laser studies have involved blocked arteries in the legs. These vessels are relatively straight and pose fewer technical problems than laser surgery on the coronary arteries. Recently, however, researchers have started using lasers to unclog coronary arteries, too. More work must be done before these procedures can be used on human patients, but they appear promising. Given the advances in both life-style moderation and medicine of the last thirty years, we can foresee conquering heart attacks, too.

ACKNOWLEDGMENTS

The creation of any book inevitably calls upon numerous people and resources and this has been no exception. While it is not possible to list all those institutions and individuals who have made this book possible, there are some whose contributions merit special recognition.

First and foremost, I want to thank my colleagues at the Alton Ochsner Medical Foundation and Ochsner Clinic for providing the time and motivation to write this book, which is in keeping with this institution's dedication to public education and preventive medicine. Dr. William Kannel not only coined the term "factors at risk," but he and his colleagues at the Framingham Heart Study have shown the nation and the world just how important it is to identify and modify these risk factors. The National Institutes of Health warrants special recognition for its national education programs in both high blood pressure and cholesterol, which have raised the public's awareness of their importance. The American Heart Association also merits recognition for its untiring efforts to educate the public about cardiovascular diseases and their prevention.

Past and present associates—Drs. Edward D. Freis, Irvine H. Page, and Harriet P. Dustan, among many others—have offered ongoing support and inspiration. Finally, but certainly not least, the many patients and their families whose experiences are recounted in this book have my heartfelt thanks and best wishes.

INDEX